SPEECH THERAPY
AND THE
BOBATH APPROACH TO CEREBRAL PALSY

Second Printing

SPEECH THERAPY
AND THE
BOBATH APPROACH
TO CEREBRAL PALSY

By

MARIE C. CRICKMAY, M.A., L.C.S.T.
Speech Therapist
Gorge Road Hospital
Rehabilitation Centre
and
Veterans' Hospital
Victoria, B. C. Canada

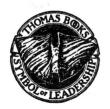

CHARLES C THOMAS • PUBLISHER
Springfield • Illinois • U.S.A.

Published and Distributed Throughout the World by
CHARLES C THOMAS • PUBLISHER
Bannerstone House
301-327 East Lawrence Avenue, Springfield, Illinois, U.S.A.
Natchez Plantation House
735 North Atlantic Boulevard, Fort Lauderdale, Florida, U.S.A.

First Printing, 1966
Second Printing, 1970

*With THOMAS BOOKS careful attention is given to all details of
manufacturing and design. It is the Publisher's desire to present books that are
satisfactory as to their physical qualities and artistic possibilities and
appropriate for their particular use. THOMAS BOOKS will be true to those
laws of quality that assure a good name and good will.*

Printed in the United States of America
R-4

to

Karel and Berta Bobath

PREFACE

THE Bobath approach to cerebral palsy is not a new one. It was gradually evolved by Mrs. Bobath in the course of her work with cerebral palsied children as far back as 1947. Since that time, the techniques of inhibition and facilitation of different levels of motor behaviour have been refined and developed, and this process is still continuing. Since its first inception it has been slowly gathering momentum, and an increasing number of people in different countries of the world want to know and understand more about it. In particular, there has been evidence of a growing desire to know more about the role of the speech therapist in this approach. What does she do? How does she integrate her work with that of the physical therapist and the occupational therapist? As there has been little published on this subject, the author, having been lucky enough to have studied and worked with Dr. and Mrs. Bobath, felt it incumbent on her to attempt to supply this information.

It is felt that, apart from their treatment, one of the major contributions of Dr. and Mrs. Bobath has been in helping to break down the artificial barriers which have existed for too long between the disciplines of physical therapy, occupational therapy and speech therapy. This book then is offered to all therapists in the hope that it will stimulate them to learn more about disciplines other than their own, and to seek ways of integrating their therapies. There is little doubt that the person who benefits most from this broader approach is—the patient.

A grateful acknowledgment is made to Dr. and Mrs. Bobath for their generosity in supplying material, and in particular to Mrs. Bobath for her help in relating speech to physical therapy.

Most sincere thanks are extended to Dr. Charles Van Riper, who not only insisted that this book should be written, but also gave invaluable advice and encouragement.

MARIE C. CRICKMAY

CONTENTS

ILLUSTRATIONS

SPEECH THERAPY
AND THE
BOBATH APPROACH TO CEREBRAL PALSY

Chapter I

A SURVEY OF THE PROBLEM

D URING the last ten to fifteen years the words "cerebral palsy" have gradually penetrated the consciousness of the general public. Slowly a growing number of people have become aware that among the mass of humanity a certain number of individuals are "different" from the rest. Usually they do not know the reason for this difference, but the outward signs of it are only too obvious. In the busy city streets the adult cerebral palsied victim, with his uncoordinated and precarious gait, his exaggerated arm and hand movements, and his facial grimaces, is at once apparent. Whereas in the past this condition might have aroused antipathy or even ridicule, now the average passer-by recognizes him as a sufferer from cerebral palsy and feels only sympathy. Cerebral palsied children, perhaps, may be seen driving through the streets in special buses on their way to the local Cerebral Palsy Clinic. These clinics, often started by the parents of these children, and at first supported largely by voluntary donations, are appearing in increasing numbers throughout the North American continent, in England and in Europe, for there is a growing awareness that the cerebral palsied child must, at least, be given a fair chance.

Our concern here is to discuss as fully and objectively as possible the kind of treatment that he is being given in these clinics. We need to ensure that in the light of our present knowledge and understanding of the problem of cerebral palsy, he is receiving the therapy that will best answer his needs and fulfill his latent possibilities.

When cerebral palsied children were first treated, the prob-

3

lem, understandably enough, was seen primarily as one calling for physical therapy. The basis of the child's disability seemed that he could not move his body in a normal way, and the physical therapist was the obvious person to deal with such a condition. Gradually it was realized that other related problems stemmed from this one basic difficulty. If, during the first year of his life, a child is unable to lift up his head, to look around, reach out for an object, to acquire hand-eye coordination, to sit up and to explore his environment by crawling, his mental development will inevitably be retarded. For in the normal child mental growth and motor development follow each other step by step. Even if his physical handicap is not sufficiently severe to retard his mental development, it is likely to restrict his field of experience sufficiently to keep him psychologically immature for his age. It came to be realized that his mental and psychological needs were as important as his physical needs. Cooper (16) expresses this belief in these words: "We often forget that we are dealing with people and not merely an aggregate of disabilities and deformities. These children have ideals and emotions like other children, and like them need a sense of self-worth and accomplishments." To help supply these needs, the occupational therapist and the speech therapist joined the physical therapist to create a rehabilitation team. The occupational therapist teaches the child the basic skills of feeding, dressing and looking after himself as far as he is physically able. The speech therapist helps him to speak. In view of the fundamental urge of human beings to communicate with each other, the work of the speech therapist inevitably assumes considerable importance. In later years, in many cerebral palsy clinics this team of three has been joined by the psychologist, the social worker, and the teacher, all working under the guidance of an orthopedic surgeon and pediatrician.

This, then is the team of workers that attempts to give the cerebral palsied child a chance to overcome his handicaps, and to live as normal a life as possible. However, before discussing the different types of therapy that are given in these clinics, it would be as well for us to clarify first, what is meant by the term "cerebral palsy," and second, to describe the physical, mental and speech characteristics of the cerebral palsied child.

WHAT IS CEREBRAL PALSY?

Abbott (1) defines this disorder as a neurological disability caused by a lesion in the motor centers of the brain. This brain damage results not only in a loss of functional muscular control, but also in sensory disturbances. Perlstein (69) believes that the term "cerebral palsy" has no specific meaning, but can be used in a general way to indicate that "some injury or damage to a person's brain has resulted in a difficulty in control of movements." Westlake (87) writes "Cerebral palsy is not a single type of neuromuscular disorder, but a group of disturbances which occur as a result of involvement of cortical or subcortical motor control areas." The Bobaths (7) describe it as a "sensorimotor disorder," and point out that it is not one condition but a group of conditions, the result of abnormal brain development or brain damage.

It can be seen that there is much general agreement in these various definitions of this disorder. The term "cerebral palsy" has come to be recognized as a general one covering a variety of specific disorders. However, these specific disorders have one characteristic in common. They are all caused by damage to the motor centres of the brain, manifesting themselves in a loss of motor control. A cerebral palsied child is just not able to move his body in a normal way. With this definition in mind, let us now discuss the different types of cases that are covered by the term "cerebral palsy."

CLASSIFICATION OF CASES

It is generally agreed that it is hard to make a clear-cut classification of cases of cerebral palsy for many of them are of a mixed character. A patient whose predominant difficulty is athetosis may, at the same time, show symptoms of spasticity. This may also occur with cases of ataxia. On the other hand, there are some cases of pure spasticity.

The manner in which spasticity or athetosis is distributed throughout the body is one means of classification. The term "monoplegia" is used to describe the spasticity or athetosis of one limb; "diplegia" the spasticity or athetosis of both upper or lower limbs; "paraplegia" the involvement of both legs; "quadriplegia" the involvement of all four limbs. "Hemiplegia" refers to the involvement of one side of the body, either the right or the left. In addition, Wyllie (90) suggests a classification based not only on the distribution of the disorder throughout the body, but also on its functional effects. According to his classification there are five main types of cerebral palsy. These are *"spasticity," "athetosis," "ataxia," flaccidity,"* and *"mixed types."* In this context, however, we can confine our discussion mainly to spasticity and athetosis, for the majority of cases requiring speech therapy are likely to fall into one of these two categories. In fact, Phelps (70) believes that athetoid and spastic cases make up more than 80 per cent of all cerebral palsy.

The Spastic Patient

The individual suffering from spasticity shows an increase in muscle tension, or muscle tone (the latter term will be used in the following pages) due to a lesion in the pyramidal tracts, that is, in the motor pathways leading down from the cortex, which govern voluntary movements. The Bobaths (8) state that this increase in muscle tone can vary from a mild degree to a state of decerebrate rigidity, depending on the exact site of the lesion, and the extent of the involvement of the extrapyramidal system. They continue this description of spasticity by writing, "In addition there is a loss of voluntary movements together with a return to a lower level of integration, with primitive synergic patterns of movement." This refers to the fact that in a spastic patient the normal patterns of movement are replaced by mass-reflex action of either the flexor or extensor type. For instance, if such a patient attempts to flex (that is, to bend) any one part of his body, such as his spine, arms or legs, he will be unable to do so without having his whole body flex. In the same way, if he attempts to extend, (that is, to stretch out) any one part of his body, this attempt will cause his whole body to extend. These primitive mass-reflex movements are typical of the spastic individual, and the more spastic he is, the more primitive are his patterns of posture and movement. Bobath (4) points out that fundamentally all spastic patients show the same abnormal postural patterns. For instance, if they lie in a supine position (that is, on their backs) they all show strong extensor spasticity. They draw back their heads and shoulders, extend their hips, knees and ankles with an inward rotation, and sometimes even cross their legs. The feet are also turned inwards. The arms may be flexed at the elbows, or the arm to which the face is turned may be extended, due to the influence of the assymmetrical tonic neck reflex.

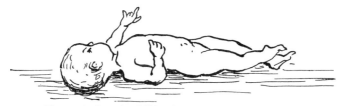

Figure 1. Spastic child lying in a supine position.

If spastic patients lie in a prone position (that is, on their stomachs) they all show strong flexor spasticity. The muscles of the neck, trunk, upper limbs and sometimes the hips, all flex, causing the spine to be rounded, the arms to be bent and often drawn in under the chest. This pattern of total flexion prevents the patient from lifting his head, extending his spine, arms and hands, and so getting onto his hands and knees. Incidentally, the spastic child very much dislikes lying in a prone position, for in it he is unable to lift his head and to move it about, or to use his arms and hands.

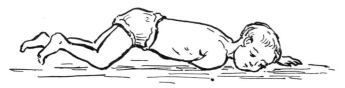

Figure 2. Spastic child lying in a prone position.

In classifying cerebral palsy according to both its distribution and its function, we describe spasticity that is present only in the two arms as "spastic diplegia." If it is present in all four limbs it is described as "spastic quadriplegia," and if it is in the right side of the body only it is classified as "spastic right hemiplegia." It is generally agreed that cases of spasticity make up about 40 per cent of all cases of cerebral palsy.

The Athetoid Patient

Athetosis is the result of a lesion in the basal ganglia. Athetoid patients show the same abnormal postural patterns as the spastic patient; that is, in the supine position their mass-reflex pattern will be predominantly of the extensor type, while in the prone position it will be predominantly of the flexor type. As the Bobaths (10) point out, these patterns are "complicated by an overlay of involuntary movements." These movements appear as a series of twisting worm-like movements, progressing from proximal to distal areas in waves, that is, they originate in the parts closest to the mid-line of the body and travel outwards to the parts furthest away from it. Phelps (70) describes the movements of severe athetoids as resembling "a nonswimmer thrashing about in the water." In addition, the athetoid shows a fluctuating muscle tone varying from hypertonicity to hypotonicity, that is, from extreme muscle tension to extreme muscle flacoidity. He alternates abrupt and misdirected movements with the rigid postures of the spastic, but unlike the spastic, he only maintains these postures fleetingly. Research shows that athetoid patients make up about 40 per cent of cerebral palsy cases.

The Ataxic Patient

Ataxia is the result of a cerebellar lesion, and it shows itself in a lack of balance and coordination. The Bobaths (10) believe that pure ataxia is rarely found among cases of cerebral palsy. In pure ataxia, muscle tone is permanently subnormal, causing the movements to become very uncontrolled. However, in many cases which are often classified as "ataxic" (but which in reality show a mixture of athetosis and ataxia), the muscle tone fluctuates from hypertonicity to hypotonicity.

These then are the physical characteristics of the main types of cerebral palsy. However, in order to get a better rounded picture of the individual patient it is also necessary to discuss his mental and speech abilities.

THE INTELLIGENCE OF THE CEREBRAL PALSIED

Evans (22) makes the following plea on behalf of the victims of cerebral palsy: "It should be strongly emphasized that cerebral palsy is not necessarily accompanied by mental deficiency or feeble-mindedness. The child's face may be expressionless, and he may drool saliva—not because he is mentally deficient, but because his muscles do not perform their normal function." Evans (23) goes on to point out that since the condition is due to brain damage it is natural that if there is too much of this injury the intelligence will be affected, this being particularly the case if the damage is in the cortex. According to his estimates 50 per cent of cerebral palsied individuals are of average intelligence, 5 to 10 per cent are exceptionally bright, 10 per cent are low grade morons, and the rest are borderline cases. Van Riper (82) states that research has shown that only about 30 per cent of cerebral palsied children are feeble-minded, and that the other 70 per cent may range all the way upward to genius level. In other words, this latter group represents a normal cross section of humanity. It is, however, extremely hard to measure a cerebral palsied child's intelligence, for the usual tests call either for some speech, or some degree of muscular coordination which is often beyond his capacity. Bobath (4) makes the point that it is particularly hard to assess the intelligence of a severely handicapped child "whose inability to respond is not necessarily due to a lack of inate intelligence, but is due in many cases to the persistence, in abnormal strength, of primitive patterns of posture and movement, which prevent more mature motor responses from making their appearance." It would be impossible for such a severely handicapped child, no matter how inately intelligent he might be, to show the same rate of mental growth and development as the normal child.

We now have a general picture of the range of intelligence of the cerebral palsied child. It is hard to over-emphasize the importance of his inate mental abilities for they will largely determine his response to therapy. This is particularly the case if he has speech problems. A severely handicapped cerebral palsied child with a low intelligence quotient may be quite unable to acquire speech, whereas a child with a similar physical handicap, but with an inately high intelligence is more likely to overcome his difficulties and learn to speak. In this connection it is interesting to note that in working with cerebral palsied children, Hood, Shank and Williamson (43) point to the imperfect relationship that exists between the severity of the affliction and the adequacy of speech and other motor skills. Carlson (13) also observes "I realized that the severity of the physical handicap was a poor criterion of the spastic's fate, and that a study of his behaviour in relation to the structural brain defect gave a much better idea of the prospect of helping him." In other words, in working with cerebral palsied individuals therapists must not judge the patient entirely by his physical handicaps, for his innate intelligence, and the environmental factors (which will be discussed later on) are at least of equal importance. With this concept in mind, let us now discuss the cerebral palsied patient from the point of view of his speech.

THE SPEECH OF THE CEREBRAL PALSIED

Approximately 65 per cent of cerebral palsy cases have some degree of speech difficulties varying all the way from slight articulatory errors to a total inability to move the speech organs sufficiently to say any intelligible words. In an attempt to study the possible distribution of these speech problems Hopkins, Bice and Colton (44) checked 1,293 cerebral palsy children. Of these they found that 64.9 per cent were quadriplegics, and that most of the speech problems were confined to this group. (It is interesting to note that this is borne out by Hoberman and Hoberman (41) who observe that many hemiplegic and diplegic children have essentially normal speech.) In this same study it was also found that 13 per cent of the children had hearing losses and 27.7 per cent had defective vision.

As could be expected, the type of speech difficulty is largely determined by the particular type of cerebral palsy. For instance, the spastic patient, with his excessive muscular tension and his sudden spasms, tends to produce speech that is explosive and punctuated by long pauses. This is what is usually referred to as "cerebral palsy" speech. In cases where there is severe speech involvement the spastic may become completly "blocked", and unable to move his speech mechanism. The athetoid patient with his overlay of involuntary movements produces speech that is extremely variable. Mild cases may show only slight articulatory errors, while severe ones may be unable to speak at all. Hoberman and Hoberman (41) observe that lack of head control, inability to swallow, with resultant drooling, add to the speech problems of athetoids. Van Riper (82) notes that in cases where there are symptoms of both spasticity and athetosis the articulation is apt to be more distorted than if spasticity alone is present. The ataxic patient produces speech that is uncoordinated, slurred and lacking in rhythm.

A great deal of research has been carried out on the differences between the speech of spastic and athetoid patients. Wolfe (89), in a study of fifty cases of cerebral palsy, related one of his tests to the "understandability" of the speech. He used this term to refer to intelligibility—how well the meaning of the passage spoken could be understood by the listener. As a result of this test, he found that 40 per cent of the athetoids could not be understood, whereas 72 per cent of the spastics had some degree of intelligible speech. Wolfe explains that these results are not altogether surprising since in a prior examination of the subjects' speech mechanism (consisting of an examination of the tongue, lips, mandible, velum, larynx and respiration) it had been found that 100 per cent of the athetoid subjects had an involvement of each organ examined, with consequent inadequate articulation. The spastic group, on the other hand, had the smallest percentage of subjects with involvement of the different speech organs, and the largest percentage of subjects having normal speech.

Research on the differences in pitch between athetoid and spastic patients has not always produced agreement. Some have found that the pitch of a spastic's speech is higher than an athetoid's," while others have found the reverse. However, many investigators, such as Duffey (20), Leith and Steer (56), and Clement and Twitchell (15) are agreed that athetoids show greater deviations, with sudden and uncontrolled changes of pitch, than spastics. Irwin (50) in a study of the mastery of speech sounds finds that there is no strong statistical evidence that differences exist between the two groups, and Byrne (12) also finds no significant differences.

These somewhat conflicting results point to the extreme difficulty of making a detailed assessment of the cerebral palsied child's speech. Indeed, it is often impossible because his speech, or lack of it, is not constant. It varies continually with the degree of his spasticity at any given moment, which itself is partly controlled by the position of his body in space at that particular moment, and partly by the amount of stimulation he is receiving from his environment. These factors are, of course, extremely variable, so that at one moment a certain speech characteristic is evident, while at the next it has disappeared and its place is taken by another. This bears out the Bobaths' belief that in working with the cerebral palsied it is necessary to see their problem in its totality, and not to isolate any one part of it. If, for instance, we attempt to isolate the speech and examine it independently of his general motor behaviour we cannot get a true picture of his speech problem. We need to view his speech behaviour in relation to the abnormal motor behaviour of the rest of his body.

We have given a brief clinical picture of the physical, mental and speech characteristics of the cerebral palsied child. Now let us consider some of the different types of therapy he is given in the many different clinics of the world. Some of these therapies are "older" and some are "newer" and, as we shall see, they have a few similarities and a few important differences. These are some of the better known.

Phelps' Muscle Re-education

Phelps was possibly the first to bring the plight of the cerebral palsied into the open. He framed the term "cerebral palsy," which is now universally accepted, and through his pioneer work in this field created a greater awareness of this problem. In all probability, many clinics throughout the world are still following his method of treatment. This is based on a detailed analysis of the muscle function of the cerebral palsied patient. Individual muscles are tested, and a careful inventory made as to whether they are spastic, flaccid, rigid or normal. Progress in treatment is assessed in terms of improvement of function of the individual muscles. In a description of his method, Abbott (1) observes that the physical therapist and the occupational therapist work closely together, in that the latter translates the control "learned in physical therapy into active feeding and dressing skills."

The Resistance Technique

In this type of therapy, associated with Kabat and Knott (54), proprioceptive stimuli are used for the development of movements which approximate the normal. These stimuli, consisting of stretch, maximal resistance and pressure, are given manually by the therapist as a means of stimulating the motor cortex. The therapy is based on the belief that these stimuli produce the maximal activation of the entire motor pathway. If weakness is apparent in both the flexor and extensor muscles, both are given heavy resistance, particularly the weaker of the two. This technique is carried out first in simple motions and then in more complicated ones, with the resistance being continually reduced. It is also applied in speech therapy. Hoberman and Hoberman (41) describe its use in strengthening the tongue protrusion and elevation. "The clinician may grasp the tongue with a piece of gauze and push back and downward . . . then the patient is instructed to push his tongue out and up as the clinician resists this movement." This method can also be used in the correction of faulty breathing patterns.

Treatment by Relaxation

The spastic and athetoid patients with their abnormally high muscle tone, sudden spasms and uncontrollable involuntary movements are obvious candidates for relaxation, and many attempts have been made to use it therapeutically. Jacobson's (51) method of progressive relaxation is probably the best known. Here relaxation is produced first by inducing its opposite, contraction, and then gradually training the patient to achieve a conscious relaxation of his muscles and muscle groups. Relaxation therapy is always carried out under favourable environmental conditions, with all stimulation reduced to the minimum. Passive relaxation techniques are sometimes used with the therapist making the movements for the patient. It is often used in speech therapy. In fact, Evans (23) writes: "Someone has said that there are three ways to treat the speech of the spastic paralytic: firstly, relaxation; secondly, relaxation, and thirdly, *relaxation.*" He agrees that this is not too easy to achieve, but notes that the best method that he has found is an adaptation of an East Indian system. In this system the clinician refers to various muscle groups, and describes a state of passivity in each of them as the patient concentrates on creating that condition.

The "Brushing" Technique

Rood (73) has developed a therapeutic technique to provide proprioceptive stimulus for the establishment of more normal motor patterns of behaviour. In the field of speech therapy she advocates a gentle stroking (either with the finger or a small dry paint brush) of the tongue or velum, in order to stimulate these areas to respond more adequately. This same technique is applied to physical therapy.

The Bobath Approach

This approach is based on the belief that, owing to the brain damage the inhibitory control, normally exerted by the higher centres of the central nervous system, fails to develop. Depending on the exact site of the lesion the cerebral palsied child will show analagous primitive reflex patterns of posture and movement. But, whereas, in normal development primitive reflexes, through the increasing use of inhibition, are broken up, elaborated and resynthetized into more mature motor patterns (increasingly under voluntary control), in the cerebral palsied child they remain constant and static, completely dominating his motor behaviour. For example, if he lies in a supine position his neck, shoulders, spine, hips, legs and feet will automatically extend, while his arms flex; and this reflex pattern of movement is so strong that he is unable to move out of it. If he lies in a prone position his neck, shoulders, arms, spine and possibly his hips will automatically flex, and again he is trapped in this one position, and unable to move.

Bobath therapy, as Mysak (64) points out "is fundamentally a tactile-proprioceptive approach designed to actualize the frequently unmanifested, but potentially present, higher motor mechanisms." Believing that it is possible to influence the central nervous system externally, the *first* aim of the treatment is to handle the cerebral palsied patient in such a way that his abnormal muscle tone becomes normalized for, as the Bobaths (10) note "muscle tone of moderate intensity forms the background against which normal movement takes place." By various means, which will be discussed later on, the abnormally high muscle tone of the spastic is reduced, while the fluctuating tone of the athetoid and ataxic patient is stabilized. The *second* aim of therapy is to inhibit the primitive reflex patterns of motor behaviour shown by the patient. Since he is unable to do this for himself, initially the therapist carries out this inhibition for him, but as soon as possible he takes over the control for himself. The *third* aim of the therapy is to facilitate the next step in the normal motor developmental process. Again, in the initial stage the therapist facilitates the more mature movement, but the patient slowly acquires the ability to perform the movement for himself. In this approach occupational and speech therapy are based on exactly the same principles as the physical therapy, and all three therapists work in close cooperation. We will be discussing the work of all three in greater detail in later pages.

SIMILARITIES IN THE THERAPIES

Similarities in the treatment of cerebral palsy can be found more easily among the "newer" therapies than between the newer and the older and more conventional methods of treatment. This can be attributed to the fact that the concepts underlying these newer therapies appear to have greater homogeneity than before. These concepts are based on a recognition that in cerebral palsy the brain lesion has caused neurological deficits which result in abnormal neuromuscular patterns of movement. There are also greater similarities in the methods of treatment among the newer therapies. More attention is being paid to the teaching of patterns of posture and movements rather than to the exercising of muscles and joints. In addition, as Bobath (4) observes: "The importance of teaching movements in the developmental sequence, that is, in the order in which they develop in the growing normal child, is more and more recognized."

There also seems to be a growing recognition that the work of the therapists should be more closely integrated. At one time it seemed that the work of the physical therapist and the speech therapist, for instance, were carried out more or less independently of each other. Each pursued her own particular approach to the problem, and although lip-service was paid to the "team-work" in a clinic, in reality little existed. More recently, however, the importance of integrating their work has become more widely recognized. As we have seen in the Kabat, Rood and Bobath approach to cerebral palsy, the principles underlying the work of the physical therapist and the speech therapist are exactly the same. Needless to say, this makes for more effective treatment.

DIFFERENCES IN THE THERAPIES

The differences between the various therapies appear to be more obvious than the similarities. The older and more conventional types of cerebral palsy treatment are based on the belief that the lesion has caused static brain damage, the effects of which cannot be mitigated or influenced in any way. Accordingly, as Mysak (64) observes, "treatment is primarily designed to help the child make the best possible use of his abnormal motor patterns." The normal motor developmental process is not followed in treatment, and instead the child is trained to sit, stand, walk (if this is at all possible) and to perform as many functional skills as he can. To achieve this he is given the help of special devices, such as braces, special chairs, standing tables and "walkers." In short, in this approach the environment is adjusted to the child's abnormal motor patterns, whereas, in the newer therapies the child is trained, as far as possible, to adjust to his environment. In view of the concept on which this older approach is based, that is, on the fundamental impossibility of alleviating the effects of the lesion, the abnormal manner in which motor skills are performed is accepted and looked upon as inevitable. As a natural result of the continued use of abnormal motor patterns bone deformities very often develop, so that orthopedic surgery is closely allied to this type of treatment.

The Bobaths (5) also take issue with the therapies that are focussed on muscle testing and the improvement in function of individual muscles. They believe that in cerebral palsy the problem is not one of muscular weakness or paralysis for, as they point out, a muscle can be too weak to contract in one position of the body, but in another it can be made to contract very strongly. For example, a cerebral palsied child may be unable to extend his elbow when his head is turned away from his arm, but he may extend the elbow easily when the head is turned towards the arm. The Bobaths believe that the problem in cerebral palsy is not one of individual muscle function, but of an impairment of coordination of muscle action. Muscles, as Bobath (3) points out, are grouped in coordinated action patterns, some contracting, some holding and others relaxing. The emphasis in this approach is on improving the function of these coordinated action patterns rather than on improving the function of individual muscles.

THE NEED FOR ADEQUATE PHYSICAL THERAPY

As we have already seen, there is a close relationship between motor development and mental development. The physical and mental horizons of the normal child broaden together, step by step, for as the scope of his physical abilities increases, so his interest in his environment grows. This is not the case with the cerebral palsied child. However, innately intelligent he may be, and as we have seen approximately 60 per cent to 70 per cent may have the normal range of intelligence, his inability to move will inevitably affect his mental development. If he is severely handicapped, and does not overcome this disability at an early age, his mental retardation may in time become indistinguishable from mental deficiency. This makes the need for adequate physical therapy an urgent one. We need to ensure that cerebral palsied children are being given the best possible treatment, so that they have a chance of fulfilling some of their potential. We believe that too many cases are being given what can only be termed as "custodial care," that is, they are being looked after

but that is all. It is well understood that severely handicapped
cerebral palsied children are unlikely to be able to earn their
living in the normal way as adults. With adequate therapy,
however, they have the possibility of being able to work in
sheltered work-shops. If they can reach this level they can lead
more normal lives and have the satisfaction of feeling they are
making some contribution to society.

THE NEED FOR ADEQUATE SPEECH THERAPY

Concomitant with the need for adequate physical therapy
is the need to ensure that we are giving cerebral palsied children
the best possible speech therapy. Again, as with physical therapy,
it is unlikely that the cerebral palsied child with a severe speech
involvement will be able to take his place in our present over-
verbal society. As Gratke (33) and Evans (24) point out, normalcy
is not our aim in these cases. The fine movements and coordinations necessary in normal speech may always be beyond the
capacity of the severely cerebral palsied child. At least therapy
should be directed towards helping the child to acquire sufficient
speech to be able to make his needs known. This, of course, is the
common aim of all types of speech therapy with cerebral palsied
children, but the means of achieving this aim differ. We feel
that these differences are related to the different concepts underlying the older and newer therapies. Speech therapy that is
based on the concept that it is impossible to mitigate in any way
the effects of the brain lesion is ready to accept the wildly
abnormal speech attempts of the severely cerebral palsied child.
It is felt that these are, at least better than nothing. When
listening to these speech attempts, which are usually accompanied
by violent movements of the whole body, we are tempted to
wonder if this is truly the case. The desire to speak is often so
strong that it produces muscle spasms which contort the child's
face and very often prevent him from making any sound at all.
This type of speech therapy can only frustrate the child, for
even at its best, his speech is often impossible to understand.

Speech therapy, however, that is based on the concept that it
is possible to mitigate, in some measure at least, the effects of the
brain lesion, can give the cerebral palsied speech that is under-

standable. Abnormal speech accompanied by movements of the body is not accepted, and the child is gradually trained to dissociate the movements of his speech mechanism from those of his body. To be most effective speech therapy has to be looked on as part of the total therapy picture, and the principles on which it is based need to be the same as those underlying the physical and occupational therapies. Given this three-fold approach, the unmanifested but potentially present, higher mechanisms of speech may have an opportunity to become actualized.

Chapter II

PRINCIPLES OF BOBATH THERAPY

WE will now discuss the principles of the Bobath approach, bearing in mind that the therapy, whether it be physical, occupational or speech, is based firmly upon them. In this approach, treatment always begins on the level at which normal development is blocked. This being the case, the first aim of the therapist, whatever her particular field, is to make a careful observation of the patient. She needs to observe his motor behaviour in particular, but also his social, psychological and speech behaviour, for the sum total of these will give her some idea of the kind of person he is. She must have this knowledge, and as much understanding of him as possible if her treatment is to be successful.

THE DEVELOPMENTAL SEQUENCE IN TREATMENT

In this approach, the cerebral palsied child's motor behaviour is always studied and related to the normal child's motor behaviour. The Bobaths (10) believe that disregard of the developmental sequence of movement patterns is often the reason for the development of deformities and contractures. In support of this they write: "Deformity appears to be the direct result of encouraging movements belonging to later stages, before the patients are able to control the motor activities of earlier stages. It is, in our opinion, of great importance to teach control over movements in the proper sequence. Although not enough in itself, this may go a long way towards the improvement of motor patterns."

Therefore, at the outset of treatment, it is necessary for each therapist to assess the cerebral palsied child's motor behaviour in order to find out at what level it deviates from the motor behaviour of the normal child. To achieve this, it is necessary to find out which of his reactions are normal, which are pathological, and which are primitive, but nevertheless, normal. For example, it might be found that, put on his feet, a cerebral palsied child of one year or more tenses his whole body, flings back his head, extends his legs and attempts to stand on his toes. This would be a pathological reaction. A normal child when put on his feet will not tense his whole body and fling back his head. He will extend his legs, but he will flex his ankles so that his heels are on the ground. The inability to flex his ankles while extending his knees and hips is pathological and typical of the cerebral palsied child for, as we have already seen, his movements are controlled by mass reflex action of either the extensor or flexor type. In the same way, it might be found that if a cerebral palsied child's head is turned to the right when he is lying in a supine position, his right arm will extend while his left arm will flex. This would be due to the influence of the assymmetrical tonic neck reflex, a primitive but normal reflex, in that it is often shown by normal babies up to the age of four months, or in some cases, even later. If a cerebral palsied child showed such a posture it would be an example of a primitive, but normal, reaction.

In testing each reaction it is also necessary to find out which movement the patient is able to do voluntarily, both with and without emotional stimulation, and which he can only do involuntarily, or merely as a reflex movement in response to a stimulus. It is important to take emotional stimulation into account in making this assessment, for a child may be able to make a movement in one situation and yet not be able to make it in another, depending entirely on the degree of emotional stimulation he is receiving. Building up a child's tolerance of disturbing external stimuli is an integral part of the therapy in each of the three fields.

Normalizing Muscle Tone

Having made an assessment of the cerebral palsied child's motor behaviour the therapist is in a position to start treatment at the level at which his development is blocked. The first step in therapy is the normalizing of the patients' muscle tone.

Sherrington (79) has said that muscle tone should be high enough to allow for the maintenance of posture against gravity, but not so high as to offer undue resistance to any intended movement. The abnormal muscle tone of cerebral palsied individuals does not fulfil these functions. In cases of spasticity, as we have already seen, muscle tone is abnormally high. In severe cases, patients show typical postures and movements, which either cannot take place at all, or can only be performed with great effort against the resistance of the increased tone. In athetosis and ataxia the muscle tone may fluctuate all the way between hypertonicity and hypotonicity. Or, in milder cases, it may fluctuate between normality and strong hypotonicity, or again, between normality and hypertonicity depending upon the degree of emotional stimulation. For example, in situations where the stimulation is within their tolerance level, these cases may show fairly normal postural and movement patterns; under conditions of over-stimulation they may revert to more primitive movement patterns. In all cases of fluctuating muscle tone, the patient is unable to stabilize and maintain bodily postures and his movements are misdirected and unpredictable.

The regulation of muscle tone throughout the body is the function of centres in the brain stem and midbrain. These centres control the muscle tone necessary for the maintenance of posture, and for the shifts of muscle tone during every voluntary movement. They also control the maintenance of equilibrium. The Bobaths (11) believe "Abnormal muscle tone is due to the release of these centres in the brain stem and midbrain from the inhibiting influence of the cerebral cortex." They believe that before a patient will be able to make normal movements it is both necessary, and possible, to normalize his muscle tone, *first,* by inhibiting his primitive reflex activity for him, and *second,* by training him to take over this inhibition for himself.

INHIBITORY CONTROL

It may help us to understand the basic premise of the Bobath approach to cerebral palsy if at this point we pause briefly, and discuss the inhibitory processes in a general way. We will gain a little insight into these processes if we remember that only one reaction can be expressed at any one time. As an example of this Ashby (2) writes: "In a simple animal like the Hydra there are only two possible reactions. If it is touched it may retract into a ball (defence reaction), or it may attempt to grasp the object and eat it (feeding reaction). Consequently, if it exhibits the defence reaction then there is only the feeding reaction to inhibit. If it had *three* reactions, then in exhibiting one there would be two to inhibit. If there were *ten* possible reactions then there would be nine to inhibit."

When we apply this same principle to the vast complexity of human behaviour we begin to get an inkling of the tremendous importance of inhibitory control. If only one response can be manifested at any one moment, then the infinite number of other possible responses must be inhibited. And this inhibition, we must remember, is not a passive but an active process. Sherrington (79) bears this out when he says "Desistance from action may be as truly active as the taking of action," a point that we need to remember when dealing with cases of cerebral palsy. At each level of the central nervous system we develop the possibility of making both more responses and more complex ones. These responses can only be manifested if inhibitory control is exercised from the cerebral cortex. At the lowest, the spinal level, movements are gross and predictable, involving large segments of the body. In the ascent from the spinal to the cortical, the highest level of integration of movements, we find, according to the Bobaths (11) "that movements become less widespread, less automatic and predictable. They become more variable and selective, and involve even smaller segments of the body." This evolution of motor patterns from those that are gross and automatic responses (as shown by the newborn infant) to those that are highly selective and voluntary (as shown by the ballet dancer) is due to the increasing ability to inhibit all but the required part of any movement. This inhibition of unwanted activity is as much a part of the movement as is the movement itself.

Inhibitory control then, is an integral part of normal development, but because, as Ashby (2) writes "Inhibitory processes are silent, and can only be discovered by inference," their importance might easily be overlooked. Our eye, naturally enough, is caught by what a person is doing. It is only by giving the matter our attention that we realize what he might have done if his processes of inhibition had not carried out their unseen work.

INHIBITORY CONTROL IN THE CEREBRAL PALSIED

In cases of cerebral palsy, however, we do see what happens when the inhibitory processes do not carry out their work. We see abnormal over-activity. The Bobaths (11) believe that this is due to the release of the lower centres of integration of postural and movement patterns from the inhibitory control of the higher centres. As a result of this release cerebral palsied patients do not possess the capacity for selective and varied movements. Instead, as the Bobaths (11) note "they are left with a few primitive reflex patterns which are stereotyped and widespread, involving the whole body in predictable synergies of muscle action." For example, as we have already seen, if a cerebral palsied child is held up and encouraged to stand on his feet he will react in either of two ways. He will either fling back his head and extend his whole body, spine, hips, knees and ankles, and attempt to stand on his toes, or, if an attempt is made to get him to flex his ankles (and stand with his heels on the ground in the normal way) he will immediately flex his knees, hips, spine, shoulders and head. In other words, he can only flex his ankles by using a reflex, the so-called *"flexor withdrawal reflex,"* which causes his whole body to flex. In the same way, he can only extend his hips and knees (as required in standing) by using another reflex, the *"extensor thrust"* which causes his whole body to extend. This inability to move any one part independently of the total pattern is typical of the cerebral palsied individual. It will be a matter of particular concern to us when we come to discuss the movements of his speech mechanism.

The patient will only be able to free himself from his primitive reflex patterns of posture and movement if his inhibitory processes can be developed. These processes, by suppressing all but the required part of any movement, will enable him to flex his ankles in standing, and yet keep his knees and hips extended. They will enable him to flex his fingers and grasp an object while keeping his wrist extended. The Bobaths (6) believe that these inhibitory processes can be developed in the cerebral palsied individual. This belief is the basic principle underlying this approach and reflex inhibition is the cornerstone of the treatment.

REFLEX INHIBITING POSTURES

The Bobaths (6) have found a way of breaking up the patient's abnormal reflex activity by a special technique of manipulation. The patient's typical postures in supine (on his back), in prone (on his abdomen), sitting, kneeling and standing are studied and analysed, and he is put into positions which are the exact reverse of these. Flexion is changed to extension, pronation to supination, adduction (movement of a limb towards the body's midline) to abduction (movement away from the midline) and vice versa. The Bobaths call these reversed postures *reflex inhibiting postures,* or "R. I. P's."

For example, let us imagine a patient whose spasticity is predominantly of the flexor type. If such a patient is placed in a kneeling position and made to sit back on his heels, his trunk will fall forward and his spine will flex. His arms will adduct and flex and his head will fall down so that it touches the supporting surface. In this position the patient is unable to extend his spine without also extending his hips and raising his trunk. He cannot extend his arms and move them forward, and there is every probability that he will be unable to raise his head.

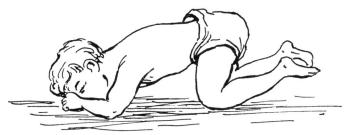

Figure 3. Spastic child in a kneeling position.

In order to effect reflex inhibition with such a patient, it is necessary to change the posture in such a way that neither the total flexion nor the total extension reflex can operate. This can be achieved by keeping the hips and knees in full flexion, and counteracting the flexion of the trunk by extending the spine, moving the arms forward and placing them on the support with full extension of the elbows, wrists and fingers. In order to counteract the inward rotation of the upper arms and the pronation of the forearms, the palms are placed facing each other. Finally, the head is raised, completing the breaking up of the flexor pattern of the upper part of the body. The total flexion of the legs (counteracting the patient's pattern of extension) is broken up by having the ankles extended.

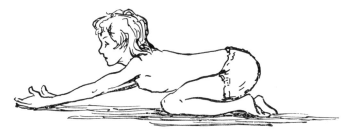

Figure 4. Heel-sitting reflex inhibiting posture.

In reflex inhibition, such as we have just described, the patient is gradually eased into the required reflex inhibiting posture, and then held by the therapist at certain "key" points. These consist mainly of the shoulder girdle, hips and spine. By holding a patient firmly and preventing reflex activity at these proximal parts, it is possible to prevent activity in distal parts of his body without actually touching these parts. In fact, with this type of manipulation it often happens that spasticity in the limbs is reduced to such an extent that the patient can move them actively on his own. For example, by guiding and controlling a cerebral palsied child from the key points it is possible to make him use his hands in sitting, and to make him crawl, stand and walk without interference from the therapist. This would not be possible, of course, with severe cases. At first it may be necessary to hold them at many points to achieve a successful reflex inhibiting posture, but soon as possible the patient is held only at the key points.

Spastics and athetoids are also handled in different ways. Severe spastics who can hardly move are not just held in a reflex inhibiting posture, but are moved within the pattern of the posture until they begin to move themselves. For instance, in the posture just described a severely spastic child might be rolled from side to side, and even right over into a supine position and back again. On the other hand, athetoids, who at all times move too much, would be required to hold a reflex inhibiting posture steadily for as long as possible. They would also be given practice in weight-bearing in these postures, in order to increase and steady postural tone.

THE EFFECT OF REFLEX INHIBITING POSTURES

At first, the patient is likely to resist being put into a reflex inhibiting posture. His abnormal posture is the familiar one and seems completely natural to him, and when the therapist begins to flex the parts of his body that previously had always been extended, and vice versa, he feels frightened and excited. Naturally enough, he struggles violently to free himslf and return to his accustomed reflex posture. He must not be allowed to do this. He must be given a great deal of reassurance and encouragement, but at the same time, he must be held very firmly during this period of mounting tension. In this connection the Bobaths (10) write: "If the reflex inhibiting posture can be maintained in spite of the struggle, the spasm gradually subsides; the patient feels easier and increasingly more comfortable in this new posture. After the spasm has died away and the patient has adjusted himself to the posture, spasticity is greatly diminished or abolished temporarily."

At first, the periods when the reflex activity has been successfully inhibited, and the patient is adjusted to the posture are only fleeting, lasting, in severe cases, for only a matter of seconds. Tension begins to build up again, resulting in another muscular spasm. Again, it is of the utmost importance that he should not be released during the spasm, for, if he were, the therapist would have failed to inhibit the spasm she had provoked by placing him into this posture. Instead, he must be held very firmly. After a relatively short time the tension will again gradually subside, and the patient will adjust once again to the new posture. Gradually, the spasms will come less frequently, and will be less severe, and the periods of adjustment, that is when reflex activity is inhibited, will last longer.

It is these periods of adjustment that are of particular interest to the therapist (whether she be a physical therapist, an occupational therapist or a speech therapist) for during it, as Marland (57) notes, a change comes over the patient's whole condition. Muscle tone throughout the whole body becomes more normal, that is, in the spastic there is diminished resistance, or absence of resistance, in the formerly spastic muscles to passive movement. Hands and fingers may open spontaneously whereas previously fingers were clenched with thumbs adducted. Breathing improves, becoming more deep and regular. In the athetoid, involuntary movements and grimacing gradually decrease, and even disappear. In the ataxic patient tremors are absent when he tries to perform a voluntary movement. Perhaps the most remarkable of all is the change that comes over the patient's face. He loses his former abnormal expression and, for the first time in his life, he looks normal. Squinting, if usually present, disappears, and focussing of the eyes becomes easier. A child who could only make rare grunts and noises sometimes, begins to babble normally and quite spontaneously. A child who could speak, but only with difficulty, is able to articulate with greater ease and clarity.

NEW PATTERNS OF SENSATIONS

The Bobaths believe that these remarkable changes are brought about by the inhibition of the patient's abnormal reflex activity, and the consequent normalization of the muscle tone throughout his whole body. For the first time in his life, as the Bobaths (11) note: "he experiences the feeling of a normal posture held by normal activity of his muscles. He receives normal sensations from his muscles and joints, and has a chance to react to these new sensations."

In the normal individual it is the proprioceptors, that is,

the group of cells that specialize in receiving stimuli from inside the organisms, that send information to the brain as to the position of the body in space, and of the position of different parts of the body in relation to each other. It is this constant flow of information from our muscles and joints that controls and guides our movements. *In a cerebral palsied child, however, the propioceptors can only send information of abnormal sensation.* The spastic with his abnormally high muscle tone feels only a heaviness in his limbs which prevents him from moving them freely and easily. His experience is limited to the feeling of lying in his habitual and abnormal postures, and moving within the limits of his reflex activity. The athetoid with his overlay of twisting, writhing movements and his fluctuating muscle tone, knows only the feeling of this condition. With reflex activity inhibited, the picture is suddenly and dramatically changed. The proprioceptors in the muscles and joints can now send normal sensations to the brain, with the result that, for the first time in his life, the cerebral palsied child experiences normal muscle tone. It is little wonder that, quite spontaneously, he immediately responds in some of the ways we have just described.

Thus the periods when he is adjusted to the reflex inhibiting posture, brief as they may be at first, are of tremendous importance to him. It is during these periods that new and normal sensory patterns of movement and posture are laid down. As the Bobaths (11) write: "The patterns of these new postures are laid down by purely sensory impressions, and without the patient's conscious attention." This is in accordance with the development of posture and movements in the normal child. The proprioceptive system conveys information to the brain as to the different positions and movements of his body, and these sensory impressions are received without his conscious attention.

THE CRITERION OF A SUCCESSFUL REFLEX INHIBITING POSTURE

We must remember that placing a cerebral palsied patient into a reflex inhibiting posture is not a guarantee that reflex inhibition will be carried out successfully. If a child is unable to adjust himself to the posture and continues to resist it, nothing has been gained. In fact, this may be a retrograde step, for his struggles may have made him temporarily even more spastic than he was before. Continued inability to adjust to a posture usually means that the patient is being placed into a posture that is too difficult for him. The postures have to be carefully graded, progressing from the easier to the more difficult ones, and they must be adapted to suit individual needs. The posture chosen must be neither too easy nor too difficult for the child. If it is too easy for him it will not produce the abnormal reactions we are wanting to inhibit, and so he will make no progress. On the other hand, if it is too difficult for him he will struggle so hard against it that he will make himself even more spastic. The patient's progress in the treatment is dependent on the skill and knowledge of the physical therapist in choosing the right reflex inhibiting posture at the right moment. This posture must be sufficiently difficult to produce an abnormal reaction, and yet not so difficult that this reaction cannot be inhibited successfully.

THE DEVELOPMENT OF SELF-INHIBITION

When the patient is first put into a reflex inhibiting posture it is the therapist who inhibits the abnormal reflex activity by holding him firmly in the posture and not allowing him to break out of it. The aim of the treatment, of course, is to train the patient to take over this control for himself. He has to learn to inhibit his abnormal reactions, that is, to give up his resistance to the posture. In order to facilitate this transition from external to internal control, the therapist begins to reduce her help. The best moment for her to begin to do this is when resistance is beginning to decrease, for at this moment the patient has a chance of taking over control for himself. Gradually the therapist holds the child less firmly. Slowly and progressively she reduces the pressure, moving her hands from one key point to another until all the help she is giving the child is, perhaps, with one finger on one key point. When he has taken full control, she is able to take her hands away altogether. However, it is necessary for her to be ready to give assistance at the first sign of tension. For after a period of adjustment, as the Bobaths (6) observe, "spasticity may recur suddenly and unexpectedly . . . particularly if the child starts to move, or moves further than he can control."

SEQUENTIAL MOVEMENT PATTERN

The inhibition of the pathological reflex activity, with the resulting reduction of spasticity, sets free the patient's potential ability to move. We have already cited an example of this in the spontaneous and normal movements made by the child when he first becomes adjusted to a reflex inhibiting posture. Movements are encouraged at every stage of the treatment, but they must be normal movements, and not the former abnormal ones. In treating the young cerebral palsied child movements are developed in the same sequence as they are acquired by the normal child. In the older patient who has already learned to sit, stand or walk, but in an abnormal way, the Bobaths (6) believe that it is necessary to go back to the early and more primitive activities which should have preceded these skills. For example, a normal baby learns to roll over onto his side, and then over into a prone position. From there he learns to get onto his hands and knees, to sit, stand and walk, each more mature movement pattern developing out of the one preceding it, and preparing the way for the one following it. The Bobaths (6) believe that it is not possible for a cerebral palsied patient to stand and walk normally if he has never acquired the earlier movement patterns. The "gaps" in his neuro-muscular development have to be filled in. He must learn to balance on his hands and knees before he will be able to balance when he stands and walks. Not surprisingly, the Bobaths (6) state that it is considerably easier to help a young child to acquire movements in the normal way than it is to fill in the gaps left in an older patient's motor development. Not only does the latter have to eradicate abnormal patterns of long standing, but psychologically, it is difficult for him to accept a return to a more infantile stage of motor behaviour.

FACILITATION OF MOVEMENTS

When a cerebral palsied patient has acquired the ability to inhibit his own reflex activity in an "R. I. P.," the next important stage in the treatment is the facilitation of normal, automatic movements. The Bobaths (6) state that these consist mainly of the fundamental righting and equilibrium reactions. They stress, however, that in their treatment the patient is not taught these automatic reactions as exercises, that is, he is not asked to perform them voluntarily. In normal development automatic movements precede voluntary ones. For example, if in the first few months of life a baby's head is turned to one side, his body turns automatically in the same direction, with the result that he will end up lying on his side. This is the result of the influence of the neck righting reflex. A few months later the picture will have changed. If he then wants to roll over into a prone position from a supine one, he will voluntarily turn his head to one side, and roll over, first, onto his side, and then over onto his front. In treating the cerebral palsied child, the Bobaths (6) believe that it is the earlier automatic righting reflexes that must first be facilitated. Later on, as with the normal child, the cerebral palsied child will be able to use these movements voluntarily.

The word "facilitation" of movements is used advisedly, for it describes exactly what takes place. The patient is moved in such a way that the righting and equilibrium reactions are all but forced to make an appearance. For example, the neck righting reflex, which we have just described, can be facilitated in the following way. With the child lying in a supine position, the therapist first flexes his head (in order to counteract the extensor spasticity) and then turns the face to the side. The child's body will then turn over onto the side to which the face is turned. By turning his head still further in the same direction, and lifting it up at the same time (in order to extend the neck and spine) the patient will roll over onto his abdomen. There are many other ways in which physical therapist can facilitate automatic reactions. For instance, she can put the patient into an uncomfortable position which, as the Bobaths (6) write "induces him to move into a more comfortable one, to right his head, and to restore the normal alignment of the head, body and limbs." Or again, she can move him in a way which necessitates automatic reactions as a protection against falling.

Equilibrium reactions are used from the first in all reflex inhibiting postures, and they are facilitated in very much the same way as the righting reflexes. For example, in sitting, kneeling and standing the patient is moved from side to side, and backwards and forwards in order to stimulate the appearance of normal, automatic balance reactions. He may be pushed slightly off balance, in order to experience the feeling of regaining it.

When movements are being facilitated in the ways we have been describing, it is necessary for the therapist to guard against the recurrence of the patient's formed abnormal reflex activity. This will be signalized by a return to his former abnormal muscle tone, and the consequent abnormality of his movements. If this occurs when movements are being facilitated, no attempt should be made to correct the movement itself, but instead it should be abandoned and the reflex inhibiting posture built up correctly once again. Only when the patient has adjusted himself to the posture again, and controlled his own reflex activity, should another attempt be made to facilitate the required automatic reactions. In this way, the cerebral palsied child is gradually trained to acquire a background of normal, basic, automatic movement patterns. Once this background has been developed, he will be able to use these movements and learn voluntary skilled movement, such as dressing and feeding himself, and later on, writing.

In a summary of the Bobath approach to cerebral palsy it could be said that the treatment consists of three stages. *First,* the pathological reflex activity has to be inhibited. *second,* the primitive but normal reflexes have to be facilitated and established. These two processes of the inhibition of lower reflexes and the facilitation of more mature patterns of neuromuscular coordination are carried out at all levels of the central nervous system starting at the lowest. From there it is carried on up to the highest level possible for the individual patient, this being dependent on the degree of his brain damage. The *third* and final stage of the therapy is the development of voluntary motor behaviour under the control of the patient.

As the Bobaths (4) state: "The treatment of all children with cerebral palsy is lengthy, and no quick results can be expected by any method." However long the treatment may prove to be with severe cases it seems that the approach we have described offers the cerebral palsied patient the best opportunity of fulfilling his potential.

Chapter III

THE TEAM APPROACH TO TREATMENT

THE three most important members of the cerebral palsy team are the physical therapist, the occupational therapist and the speech therapist. In most clinics, these three are working under the direction of an orthopaedic surgeon or pediatrician, often with the additional assistance of a psychologist and social worker. The success of such a team, as Mitchell (59) observes, depends on their ability to integrate their efforts towards achieving a common objective. Each member of the team has to realize, first, that her contribution alone could not resolve the problem, and second, that it only gathers the necessary weight and force when it is added to the total therapeutic program.

It often happens, however, that in spite of such a mutual recognition of aims, difficulties arise in the smooth operation of such a team. This, as often as not, can be attributed to the great lack of communication that ordinarily exists between the various disciplines, in this case particularly, between the disciplines of physical therapy, occupational therapy and speech therapy. If therapists from these three disciplines intend to work together successfully then it is necessary for each therapist to be able to communicate the aim and function of her work to her colleagues. Even this obvious step is often complicated by the fact that each discipline has evolved its own language of technical terms, which are often incomprehensible to the outsider. Therefore, as Neal (65) has suggested, if members of different disciplines are to work together successfully, they should be ready to teach the language of their own discipline, and at the same time, to learn the language of the others.

In the Bobath approach to cerebral palsy, however, some of these difficulties are obviated by the fact that each of the three therapists on the team will have received special training in the theory and application of this particular method. As a result, they will have a common goal in therapy, a common language, and above all, as Mitchell (59) points out, they will have acquired the capacity to think within the conceptual schemes of other disciplines. These are great advantages, and the therapists who receive such a training are fortunate in being pioneers in a field that is only just beginning to be developed. Artificial barriers between physical therapy, occupational therapy and speech therapy have existed too long. They are undoubtedly detrimental to the patient in that each therapist, working exclusively within the boundaries of her own discipline, does not see him as a whole person. This limited approach handicaps the patient's recovery and often prevents him from fulfilling his recovery potential. We believe that the breaking down of these barriers (as carried out in the Bobath approach) is a major step forward in the therapeutic field.

THE PHYSICAL THERAPIST AS THE LEADER OF THE TEAM

As cerebral palsy is primarily a sensory-motor disorder affecting the patient's ability to move his body and limbs in a normal way, the physical therapist inevitably holds the key position on the team. The progress she makes with the patient largely determines how far the occupational therapist and the speech therapist will be able to go, or indeed, whether they will be able to get beyond the initial stages of their treatment. For in occupational therapy, and even more in speech therapy, the patient must have the ability to make fine and selective movements. For example, in occupational therapy, if a child is to learn to dress himself he must be able to maintain sitting balance, and at the same time be able to move his arms and grasp an object. In speech therapy, if he is to learn to speak intelligibly he must be able to move his organs of speech without associated movements of his head, shoulders, or of the rest of his body. Whether or not the cerebral palsied patient will be able to make these fine, selective movements depends largely on the progress made by the physical therapist in her treatment. She is the one who, in the first instance, must initiate the development of the patient's latent powers of inhibition which, as we have already seen, make possible his ability to move one part of his body independently of another. At first, in severe cases, this may have to be carried out at the lower (spinal) level of co-ordination. By progressively inhibiting pathological and primitive reflex behaviour, and facilitating more mature movement patterns at higher and higher levels of the central nervous system, the physical therapist is able to bring the patient gradually to the neuro-muscular level of development required first, by the occupational therapist, and then by the speech therapist. Movements of the arms and hands, required in occupational therapy, are, of course, more gross than the movements of the jaw, lips and tongue required in speech therapy. Thus, the occupational therapist will be able to start working with the patient before the speech therapist. Following the normal developmental sequence, speech will be one of the last basic skills to be acquired by the cerebral palsied patient.

ASSESSING THE PATIENT'S MOTOR BEHAVIOUR

At the outset of the treatment the physical therapist makes a careful and detailed assessment of the patient's motor behaviour, to find out at which point his neuro-muscular development has been blocked. She is able to get this information by putting him in a number of different postures, and observing his reaction to them, and also by testing his ability to move from one position to another. For example, she observes his posture in a supine and a prone position, in kneeling, sitting and standing (if he is able to do this) ; and she also tests his ability to move from a supine to a prone position, to get onto his hands and knees, to sit, get onto his feet and, finally, to walk. From such an examination she is able to observe which of his responses are pathological, which are primitive but normal, and which are normal. Treatment begins at the point at which his reactions deviate from normal motor development.

If, after making such an assessment the physical therapist finds that the patient's neuro-muscular development is sufficiently advanced to enable him to benefit from occupational therapy and speech therapy, she will notify the two other therapists to this effect. The occupational therapist and the speech therapist then make their own assessments of the patient. These assessments are made from exactly the same standpoint as the physical therapists', that is, to establish which of the child's responses are pathological, which are primitive but normal, and which are normal. The occupational therapist assesses the child's ability to maintain sitting balance while moving his arms and hands, and his ability to grasp and release objects. She also tries to establish the maturation level of his hand-eye coordination, which will be of importance in the teaching of self-feeding, and of his perceptive abilities, which will be of importance in teaching him to dress himself. The speech therapist assesses the child's ability to move his head independently of his shoulders, which has been found to be a prerequisite for speech, and his ability to suck, swallow, chew, to produce voice, babble and say words and sentences. A detailed study of the speech therapist's assessment will be given in a later chapter.

When each therapist has made a detailed study of the child's motor behaviour in her own particular area of work, the therapists pool their information. Using the physical therapist's assessment as a basis, they are able to build up a composite picture of the child's motor behaviour from the most gross to the finest movements of which he is capable. This enables each therapist to see the child as a whole, not just from her own particular angle, and to establish at which point treatment must be started. At regular intervals throughout the course of the treatment the therapists assess their patient in order to discover if any changes have taken place in his physical condition. Again they discuss their findings with each other, so that these changes, if any, can be related to his total motor behaviour.

THE PSYCHOLOGICAL ASPECT

To assess a cerebral palsied patient's motor behaviour and nothing more would not give a true picture of his total problem. It is equally important to find out as much as possible about him as a person. If he is a child, it is necessary to get to know his parents, and to learn from them about his past history, his present environment, and the way he is reacting to it. In other words, the psychological aspects of the problem need to be given quite as much consideration as the physical aspects. In actual fact, they probably should be given greater emphasis, for in the final analysis it is the therapist's insight into the patient, and her understanding of his special difficulties that tip the balance between the success or failure of treatment. At this point, the other members of the cerebral palsy team, the physician, the psychologist and the social worker can give invaluable assistance in supplying the therapists with much necessary information. Each therapist also tries to get to know the patient for herself. Before starting treatment she spends time establishing good relations with him, for a strong rapport between therapist and patient is the cornerstone of any therapeutic situation. Again, the therapists share their impressions and insights with each other and with the other members of the team, so that among them they can add another dimension to their previous picture of the patient. When the study of both his physical and his psychological characteristics has been completed, treatment is begun.

BASIC OCCUPATIONAL THERAPY

Even if at the outset of treatment a cerebral palsied child has not sufficient control of his arms and hands to benefit from formal occupational therapy, or of his speech mechanism to benefit from formal speech therapy, there are still vital ways in which both the occupational therapist and the speech therapist can help him. This work, which needs to be carried out even with the most severely handicapped child, could be described as "basic" occupational and speech therapy. We will describe basic occupational therapy first.

This is concerned with the vital matter of teaching the mother how to handle her child physically. In this connection, Fairgrieves (25) stresses that the important factor is to teach the parents how to handle their child, as he is *now,* at the very moment of starting his physical therapy. If this basic instruction is not given, parents, naturally enough, will continue to handle their child as they always have done. In the vast majority of cases this would mean they would put him into positions that would continue to provoke the abnormal reflex activity that the physical therapist is beginning to inhibit during her sessions with the child. For example, cerebral palsied children are often dressed when lying in a supine position either across the mother's lap, or, if they are older, on a bed. This position, as we have already seen, favours extensor spasticity, and the child will react with extensor spasms, flinging back his head, arching his back and extending his hips and legs. There are two positions that will inhibit these spasms, and so make the dressing easier for the mother. The first is to put the child into a sitting position with his back to her, either on her lap, or on a stool between her legs. The second is to put him into a side-lying position on the bed, and roll him from side to side, as required. The occupational therapist explains the reason for these positions as she demonstrates them to the mother, and gets her to do it. In the same way, the therapist shows the mother how to handle the child when bathing and feeding him. Supine positions are again usually favoured by mothers for both these activities, but as soon as it is realized that they provoke spasms and abnormal reflex activity, they will be gladly discarded for ones that are easier for both mother and child. The basic postures prescribed by the occupational therapist, and endorsed by the physical therapist, will depend, of course, on the individual patient's needs. As we have already observed, all children with cerebral palsy show the same abnormal postural patterns; therefore, the positions that remedy these patterns will be similar. Their purpose needs to be explained to the mother, and her cooperation obtained in handling the child in such a way that he is not able to take up his habitually abnormal postures. The occupational therapist needs to show the mother how to bathe the child in a supine position, and yet prevent the occurrence of extensor spasticity by bringing his head and shoulders forward and flexing his hips so that his knees are on his chest.

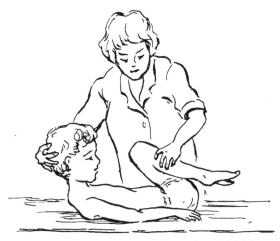

Figure 5. Cerebral palsied child in a supine reflex inhibiting posture with hips, knees, spine, shoulders and head flexed.

She also shows the mother a similar side-lying position, which is often the easiest for the child in the early stages of the treatment.

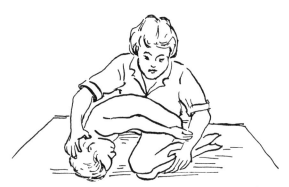

Figure 6. Cerebral palsied child in a side-lying reflex inhibiting posture with hips, knees, spine, shoulders and head flexed.

Fairgrieves (25) notes that even with a severely handicapped child a good reflex inhibiting posture, and patience until this is tolerated (which may take more than one session), can produce surprising results in the form of spontaneous, purposive movements of the arms and hands.

PLAY ACTIVITIES

There is one more brief point to be brought up in connection with basic occupational therapy, and that is the question of the cerebral palsied child's play activities. At the outset of treatment the occupational therapist may find that at home the child has been encouraged to use a tool, such as a hammer, or crayon or pencil before he is able to use it properly. In other words, his hand-eye coordination and his grasp and release mechanism are not sufficiently developed to enable him to use a tool in anything but an abnormal way. If this is found to be the case the occupational therapist gets the parents' cooperation in trying to channel the child's interest elsewhere until such a time as he reaches a higher level of neuro-muscular development. Premature attempts to use a tool will only increase the child's abnormal reflex activity, for primitive reflex movements will be the only ones available to him at that time. In the case of a severely handicapped child the occupational therapist may suggest that the parents should play *for* the child, by bringing activities to him and complying with his instructions. Naturally enough, the role of "boss" with his parents as workers is highly satisfying to the child.

BASIC SPEECH THERAPY

We have discussed ways in which the occupational therapist can help a cerebral palsied child before he is ready for more formal therapy. Let us now discuss this question from the point of view of the speech therapist.

Basic speech therapy can be given even to a severely handicapped child long before he is ready for more formal instruction. In its essence it consists of the nonverbal communication that takes place between the child and his mother. This is the forerunner of speech as it lays down the pattern of communication between the child and another person; in the first instance, his mother, but later on, other people in his environment. It starts from the moment the child is born and continues until he begins to talk, and even long after that. Its most important and fruitful period is in the first few months of life. At first, the communication is through the sense of touch. By the way she holds the child the mother is able to communicate her love and devotion to him. Gradually, as the infant develops, he becomes responsive to the sound of his mother's voice. He does not understand the words she is using, but he knows the intonations and inflections of her voice that make him feel warm and secure. He also communicates with her through *his* voice, and she is quick to understand and respond to the different needs he expresses through his crying, screams, grunts, sighs and gurgles. In a few weeks he is able to focus his eyes for the first time on his mother's face, and when she smiles at him he communicates with her by smiling back. It is not long before they begin to communicate with each other in another way. When she talks to him he begins to coo and babble answers back to her, and they "talk" together in a way that is highly satisfactory to them both.

This nonverbal communication is the foundation upon which speech is built. If the relationship between mother and child has been a satisfying one for them both, and they have communicated with each other happily and successfully, the child will take the next step of verbal communication in his stride. He will want to learn to speak in order to have more opportunities to enjoy this pleasant activity. If, on the other hand, the nonverbal communication between the child and his mother has not been a satisfying and happy experience he is likely to have difficulty in learning to speak, for the basic reason that communication is not associated with a pleasant feeling.

Basic speech therapy then, with the cerebral palsied child who has not yet learned to speak consists of two stages. First the therapist has to ensure that successful nonverbal communication has, and is still, taking place between the child and his mother. If after contact with both the mother and child she feels that their relationship is not as successful as it could be, resulting in a lack of communication between them, she should do what she can to remedy the situation. She may find that the child's physical handicap is so gross that it has prevented the mother from making contact with the child as a person. Or, it may be that the mother has not realized the importance of her relationship with the child, and the bearing that it has on his future ability to communicate. Whatever the reason, it is for the speech therapist to discuss the situation with the mother, and do all in her power to help her establish a better relationship with the child so that nonverbal communication begins to take place between them.

The second stage in basic speech therapy is to try to extend the nonverbal communication of the mother and child to include other people in the environment, particularly the speech therapist herself. The therapist needs to spend time with the child so that he gets to know her sufficiently well that he wants to communicate with her as he does with his mother. If this can be achieved, the foundation for more formal speech therapy (when the time is ripe) will have been laid.

These, then, are the ways in which the occupational therapist and the speech therapist can help the cerebral palsied child before he is ready for more formal therapy. Let us now discuss the level of neuro-muscular development he needs to have reached in his physical therapy before he will be able to start first, occupational therapy, and then speech therapy.

PRE-REQUISITE FOR SELF-FEEDING

Before the cerebral palsied child can be taught to feed himself, he must have adequate sitting balance. In this approach special chairs and other equipment, such as "walkers" are not used as it is felt that they tend to perpetuate the patient's abnormal reflex postures and movements. In this treatment, as has already been explained, the environment is not adapted to the abnormal requirements of the patient. Instead, his abnormal reflex patterns of posture and movement are inhibited, and the normal postures and movements facilitated for him. He would not be encouraged to sit in an ordinary chair until he has reached the level of neuro-muscular development that enables him to do it in a normal way. Therefore, the ability to have adequate sitting balance on an ordinary chair is looked upon as a prerequisite for self-feeding. In addition, the child's hand-eye coordination should be at least to the one year level, that is, he can pick up small objects between his finger and thumb, but he reverts to a palmar grasp on the spoon. If the physical therapist has been able to bring the child to this level in her therapy, then the occupational therapist is able to teach self-feeding. The speech therapist may also come into the picture at this point. There seems to be a strong possibility, although this has not yet been sufficiently investigated, that the child will not be able to feed himself until he is able to chew solids. The problem of teaching the child to chew will be the concern of the speech therapist, as chewing (with sucking and swallowing) is a prerequisite for speech. Therefore, the speech therapist and the occupational therapist need to work closely together at this point in the treatment.

PRE-REQUISITES FOR DRESSING

Before the occupational therapist can teach the cerebral palsied child to dress himself, he again needs to be able to maintain sitting balance. This time, as well as being able to balance, he needs to be able to move his arms, to hold the clothes with a digital grasp, and also to reach for all the necessary garments. This obviously represents a more complicated maneuver for the child. Fairgrieves (25) makes the point that athetoids often find it easier to carry out these movements when sitting on the floor, while spastics can be taught to dress while sitting on a chair. In addition to having reached the neuro-muscular level of development that makes these movements possible, the cerebral palsied child must also have reached a certain level of perception. If he is to dress himself he must know the different parts of his body, realize laterality, and how his garments are related to his body. Only when he has developed these perceptions will the occupational therapist be able to teach him to dress himself and, most important of all, teach the parents how to handle him as he learns this new skill.

TRAINING IN PERCEPTION

As soon as the physical therapist has been able to inhibit the child's pathological reflex behaviour, and is successfully facilitating more mature motor behaviour, the occupational therapist may have to begin training the child in perception. In the first twelve months of his life the normal baby gradually and unconsciously acquires, first, an image of his own body, and then an awareness of his own body in relation to his environment.

These perceptions develop naturally as the result of the ever-widening scope of his physical abilities. For example, he discovers his own hands and plays with them; he puts them in his mouth and sucks them, and then sucks anything he can lay his hands on. He learns to sit up, to get onto his hands and knees, to stand and walk. A severely handicapped cerebral palsied child, up to the time of starting his treatment has been denied these experiences. He cannot bring his hands together and play with them; he cannot pick up objects, hold them in front of him, look at them and drop them. He cannot get onto his hands and knees or sit. Therefore, he has not had the opportunity to develop the normal perceptions of a normal child, and very often he has to be taught them.

The occupational therapist's aim is to give him a stable body image, and a conception of laterality, particularly of left leading to right in preparation for reading. Progressing from simple actions requiring gross movements (such as reaching for an object) to more complicated ones requiring finer and more specific movements (such as grasping and releasing), she tries to give him an awareness of his own body in relation to his environment.

The physical therapist and the speech therapist are also interested in helping the child to develop a stable body image. An awareness of the position of his body in space, and of his limbs in relation to his body is a necessary part of normal movement, and the sooner a child develops these perceptions the more quickly he will progress in his physical therapy. In the same way, the more thoroughly the child becomes aware of himself and orientated to his surroundings, the sooner he will develop a more normal concept of himself, a concept that will include the possibility of being able to talk. Therefore, at this point in the treatment all three therapists will combine in trying to develop the child's powers of perception.

PRE-REQUISITES FOR SPEECH THERAPY

We believe that the first prerequisite for speech therapy is sufficient intelligence for speech. The child must have reached a level of mental development that indicates he is ready to learn to talk. We realize that it is not always easy to assess a cerebral palsied patient's intelligence, but from observation of his psychological behaviour, and the success or failure of the non-verbal communication that has taken place between the child and his mother, we should be able to assess it at least enough to gauge his readiness for speech. If he does not appear to have the mental ability, in spite of having the physical prerequisites for speech, therapy should be delayed. There may be some cerebral palsied children with such severe brain damage that they will never develop the capacity to speak, as there are similar noncerebral palsied children.

The second requisite for speech therapy is that the child must have reached a level of neuro-muscular development that makes it possible for him to exercise some control over the speech mechanism, and the parts of his body related to it. Speech therapy that is initiated before the patient has reached this stage of physical "readiness" can only lead to frustration and tragedy for him. This can be readily understood when it is remembered that before treatment a severely handicapped child can only make gross movements in an abnormal way. For example, if he is sitting on his mother's lap and attempts to lift his head to look at something, the effort to make this movement will immediately produce an extensor spasm and cause him to fall back with extended spine, hips and legs, and his head thrown back. How can such a patient be expected to make the fine movement of his jaw, lips and tongue, as required in speech? It is, of course, quite impossible for him, and if it is attempted it will only increase his abnormal reflex activity. For if such a patient attempts to open his mouth for speech when lying in a supine position, he would only be able to do it by flinging back his head and extending his whole body. Then his mouth would indeed be open, but only as part of the reflex movement. But then how could he close it? As long as he is in a supine position this would be impossible. If he is moved into a prone position, his flexor spasticity would become dominant. His back, head, arms would flex (and possibly even his hips) and his mouth would close, but again only as part of the total reflex movement. In that position he would not be able to open his mouth.

This, of course, refers only to severely handicapped patients. These usually consist of spastics and athetoid quadriplegics, especially those athetoids in whom the neck and arms are much more affected than the legs. Cerebral palsied patients whose legs are more affected than their arms and neck usually have normal articulation. There are also some cases whose speech is not affected at all, due to the particular site of the lesion.

CONTROL OF THE SPINE AND LOWER RIBS

From the point of view of the patient's motor behaviour, we believe that therapy should not be started until his abnormal reflex activity has been inhibited, and he is able to move those parts of his body which have some bearing on the production of speech. One such part is the spine and lower ribs, for the flexibility, or nonflexibility of these parts will determine the quality of the patient's breathing, and breathing is for speech what muscle tone is for movement, that is, it is the background for speech. Sustained tone, such as is required for the speaking of sentences, can only be obtained if the individual has the ability to emit a sustained and controlled breath. He will only be able to do this if his lower ribs are able to move in a free and normal way. When a normal individual inhales, the six lower ribs swings out in a pail-handle movement, increasing the size of the chest laterally, while at the same time the diaphragm descends, increasing the size of the chest longitudinally. In exhalation, of course, the reverse process takes place, the ribs swing back into their former position, the diaphragm relaxes and the chest is reduced to its former size.

In cerebral palsied cases, however, there are many interferences with this normal procedure. In many spastics the spine is fixed and rigid, and as a result of the release of pathological reflex activity, is held habitually in an abnormal position. This prevents the free and normal movement of the lower ribs and diaphragm. In addition, with some cases, inhalation immediately produces extensor spasticity, especially in the supine position, while exhalation produces flexor spasticity, especially in the prone position. The implication of this for speech will be discussed later.

CONTROL OF THE HEAD

Another part of the body having an important influence on the cerebral palsied patient's "readiness" for speech therapy is the head. The ability to steady and hold the head in supine lying (as a preparation for pulling up into a sitting position) seems to be another prerequisite for the development of speech. The control of the trunk and neck muscles against gravity seems to have a decisive influence on the control and coordination of the speech musculature. This can be easily understood if the important role of fixation in the performance of fine, selective movements is realized. For instance, fine and delicate movement of the fingers would be impossible without the fixation of the wrist and elbow. In the same way, fine and selective movements of the jaw, lips and tongue cannot take place without the necessary fixation of the neck and shoulders. Uncontrolled muscle action will influence all movements of the larynx, jaw, lips and tongue.

The normal baby begins to get full control of the trunk and head at six months of age. He can then hold the head in proper alignment with the trunk in sitting. He can also pull himself up into a sitting position, and lift the head for the first time in supine lying. This is the final stage of head control after having learned to lift and hold the head in prone lying at the age of two months. At seven months the child is in the full throes of babbling, that is, he is beginning to make consonant sounds that are produced by the movements of the jaw, lips and tongue, instead of just the vowel sounds he had made earlier. There may be a connection between the ability to fixate and control the head, and the ability to make fine and selective movements of the jaw, lips and tongue.

There is yet another facet of this question of head control that is of great importance to the speech therapist. It seems that when head control is established it is much easier for the patient to close his mouth, and to keep it closed for longer periods. This allows him to swallow his saliva instead of letting it pour out of his open mouth. Excessive drooling is, of course, very characteristic of these patients, and the speech therapist needs the help of the physical therapist in overcoming this problem. By helping the patient to acquire head control the physical therapist is preparing him for speech therapy.

In summarizing the way in which the team works together in this approach to cerebral palsy we observe that the physical therapist usually is the first one to work with the patient. She prepares him for occupational therapy, and then the two therapists help him to reach the stage of "readiness" necessary for speech therapy. When all three therapists are working with the patient, they keep each other informed as to the stage of therapy they have reached. For example, the speech therapist lets the occupational therapist know when she is inhibiting the sucking reflex and facilitating the chewing reflex, so that the occupational therapist can help the child to carry this new skill over into the feeding situation.

It sometimes happens that a child will produce his first sounds spontaneously with the physical therapist, or the occupational therapist rather than with the speech therapist, for the simple reason that in those situations there is no emphasis on speech. If this happens, the speech therapist advises the other therapists how to proceed and encourage the child to vocalize even more. Later on, when the child is beginning to understand the speech of others, and to put his own words together into short sentences, the occupational therapist is in an excellent position to help him. As Ellis (21) points out, she can "teach the meaning of language involving temporal and spatial relationships, such as when she asks the child to "Put it here," or "Do it now."

It also sometimes happens that the physical therapist and the speech therapist work together on a patient. The physical therapist putting him into postures, or moving him in a way that normalizes his muscle tone, while the speech therapist encourages him to babble and say words while his general condition is more normal. There is no rigid plan in this cooperation between the therapists. It develops spontaneously and naturally out of their common belief that the more their therapy is coordinated, the more the patient benefits.

Chapter IV

DEVELOPMENT OF MOTOR BEHAVIOUR AND SPEECH IN THE NORMAL AND CEREBRAL PALSIED CHILD

To understand the abnormal motor behaviour of the child suffering from cerebral palsy, it is necessary to have some knowledge of the development of motor behaviour in the normal child, for in the Bobath approach the therapy follows the normal developmental pattern step by step. A study of the development of motor behaviour entails, as Gesell and Armatruda (28) point out, an examination of the central nervous system.

There are two characteristics of the normal development of the central nervous system that have particular significance in this approach.

1. *Development follows an orderly pattern.* Gesell and Thompson (30) state that "Behaviour as it matures follows an orderly progress," so that "each stage is the outcome of the one preceding it and the prerequisite of the one following it." Griffiths (35) relates this specifically to infant behaviour by noting that "a certain orderliness exists in the way a baby develops. He must sit before he creeps, and (usually) creeps before he walks. He must vocalize and babble before he talks."

2. *Development always proceeds from the general to the specific.* Hurlock (46) has made the point that in both prenatal and postnatal development, *general* activity precedes specific activity, this being apparent first in muscular responses. "The newborn infant moves his whole body at one time, instead of moving any one part of it." Gesell and Armatruda (28) describe this developing process in the following way: "As the nervous

50

system undergoes growth differentiation, the forms of behaviour also differentiate. At one age he seizes with his fist; at a later age he plucks with neat opposition of thumb and index—a concrete example of the way differentiation produces specialization of function and new behaviour patterns." These two characteristics of the normal development of the central nervous system will be observed in the following brief description of the normal baby's motor, psychological, speech and language development from birth to three years of age.

MOTOR RESPONSES OF THE NEWBORN INFANT

In order to understand the motor behaviour of the newborn infant it is necessary to have some knowledge of reflex motor behaviour and of the way in which, as the nervous system matures, primitive reflex movement patterns are gradually modified and superseded by more complex patterns of behaviour under voluntary control. Chusid and McDonald (14) describe reflexes as "inborn stimulus-response mechanisms" and point out that the instinctive behaviour of lower animals is largely governed by reflexes. The Bobaths (11) observe that stimulation at any level of the central nervous system produces movement. At the lowest, the spinal level, the stimulation produces gross reflex movements, involving large segments of the body. In the ascent from the spinal to the cortical level these primitive movements, through progressive inhibition, are gradually broken up, discarded and resynthetized into more complex patterns of movement. At the highest cortical level, through a combination of inhibition and training, a dancer, for instance, can make a tiny, isolated movement of the fingers without an associated hand movement.

In studying the motor behaviour of the newborn infant we are not concerned with the highest level of the central nervous system but rather with the spinal and brain stem level. As we have seen, stimulation at this level produces primitive and automatic movements involving large segments of the body. For instance, if the newborn infant is startled by a sudden change of position he will automatically react with a total movement of his whole body. Or, if his head is turned to one side, his body will automatically begin to turn in the same direction. In other words, at this stage in his development his behaviour is entirely reflex in character.

At birth we find several important reflexes affecting the speech mechanism, or having some relationship with it, and these are of paramount importance in understanding the speech of the cerebral palsied.

1. *The Neck Righting Reflex* This is present at birth and serves to keep the head in line with the body. For instance, if the baby is lying in a supine position and his head is turned to one side, his body will automatically begin to turn in the same direction, thus enabling him to turn onto his side. This reflex is strongest during the first three months of life, but, as the central nervous system matures, the ability to make more isolated movements gradually develops with the result that between the sixth and tenth months this reflex becomes modified. From then on it becomes weaker and weaker, finally disappearing about the fifth year. At this age the child will have developed the ability to turn his head without any associated turning movement of his body.

2. *The Moro Reflex or "Startle" Reaction* Bobath (11) states this is a characteristic reaction of infants to "a number of stimuli, such as movement of the supporting surface, tapping of the abdomen, sudden passive extension of the legs, or blowing on the face." The reaction consists of a sudden extension and abduction of the arms, hands and fingers from their usual flexed posture followed by adduction and flexion on the chest. The legs follow the same movement pattern. This reaction is present at birth and is at its strongest during the first three months of life. Thereafter it gradually becomes weaker and less apparent, but it never completely disappears. Even an adult, if suddenly and violently startled, will show symptoms of this same reaction. This reflex may remain persistently strong in the cerebral palsied child past infancy into his older childhood.

3. *The Assymetrical Tonic Neck Reflex* In this reflex, the rotation of the head to one side leads to an increase of extensor tone in the limbs toward which the face is turned, while the opposite limbs show an increase of flexor tone. If the reflex is

strong, the arm and leg towards which the face is turned show movements of extension, while the other two members flex. The effect of this reflex in the arms is more pronounced than on the legs; indeed, it may show itself in the arms only. According to Gesell and Armatruda (28) and Schaltenbrand (76) this reflex can often be seen in infants from birth up to sixteen weeks, the head being held to one preferred side, usually the right. However, the Bobaths (9) note that the reflex is never strong, and the infant can easily take up any other attitude, and move his limbs freely regardless of the position of the head. This reflex is often over-active with children suffering from cerebral palsy. The Bobaths (9) maintain that "If the child is severely affected the assymetrical tonic neck reflex is nearly always present, with the result that the child becomes fixed in the tonic neck attitude, and the movements of the limbs are dependent on the position of the head. The reflex persists beyond the sixteenth week, and may become even stronger as spasticity increases."

The gross reflex movements that we have been describing, however, are not the only reactions that have some relationship with the speech mechanism, or with parts of the body closely associated with it, such as the head, neck and shoulders. At birth, babies show other less specific responses which also have a bearing on speech development. These will also be found in children with cerebral palsy, possibly to a greater degree, and certainly for a longer period. So if we are to understand these children we must concern ourselves with these early basic aspects of their behaviour.

During the first days of life Hurlock (46) notes that the infant focusses his eyes momentarily on a light held in front of him, but, on the whole, the eye movements are very uncoordinated. Along with these brief visual *fixations* we also find *spontaneous eye movements*. These consist of opening the eyes and rolling the eye-balls from side to side with little or no coordination at this time. *Feeding responses,* such as sucking, toothless biting, puckering, swallowing and choking also occur. These reactions are called forth by hunger, and by direct stimulation in the region of the mouth, whether it be the touch of a nipple or some object unrelated to food. We shall find them interferring with the speech of the cerebral palsied child. Perhaps belonging to the same category is the *sucking of fingers,* a reaction which has appeared as early as twenty minutes after birth. *Yawning* often occurs within the first hour after birth, and can be aroused by touching the lips and chin. We find *hiccupping* occurring during the first hours of life. Often during sleep the infant will open and shut his mouth rhythmically, and in many instances, the tongue will protrude for as much as half an inch in these *rhythmic mouthing movements.* These are often accompanied by slight *frowning and wrinkling of the brow,* also usually occurring during sleep. In the newborn we also notice movements of *turning and lifting the head.* When placed in a prone position, babies can lift their heads slightly on the very first day of life, and this ability enables them when prone to free their mouths for breathing. *Hands and arm movements* also occur. When the infant is asleep, as well as when he is awake, the arms and hands are in almost constant motion. The arms are waved around in a random, aimless fashion, and the hands open and shut for no apparent purpose. The resemblance of this early picture of the normal child to that presented by certain cerebral palsied persons of all ages is clear. The *crying* of a new-born infant is always accompanied by body movements, and the more vigorously he cries the more vigorously he uses every part of his body. In a study of speech elements during the first six months of life, Irwin (50) noted that in an analysis of over a thousand vowel sounds heard in the cries of forty new-born infants the "a" sound, as in "hat" predominated. An overwhelming majority of the crying sounds were front vowel sounds (92 per cent): middle vowel sounds were infrequent (7 per cent), and back vowel sounds were present only about 1 per cent of the time.

In trying to observe the difference between the motor behaviour of the newborn normal infant and the newborn cerebral palsied infant we must remember that, during the first few months of life, it is hard to detect signs of cerebral palsy. As the Bobaths (7) observe, at first the cerebral palsied baby, like the normal baby, shows a preponderance of flexor tone. The limbs are held in flexion and resist passive extension. It is, in fact, only when extensor tone starts to develop from about the sixth week onwards that the cerebral palsied baby begins to show signs of spasticity. The Bobaths (10) have made the point that the earliest complaint of the mother is that her baby does not use his legs to kick, as the normal baby does, or that he only kicks with one leg.

THE BABY AT ONE MONTH

We have presented a motor portrait of the baby at birth. Let us view him a month later. He is larger and less red. He has first lost and then regained his birth weight. The expression of his face is still vague. His hand will clench on contact with an object, but has to be pried open to receive a rattle, which he immediately drops. He cries and sneezes at the slightest provocation, and makes small throaty noises usually after feeding. His central nervous system is more organized than it was at birth. Gesell and Ilg (29) sum up his progress in these words: "His breathing is deeper and more regular: his swallowing is firmer. He does not choke or regurgitate as freely as he used to. He is less susceptible to startling. He begins to react positively to comfort and negatively to discomfort, and to use crying and other sign language to express his demands and desires."

His Reflex Behaviour

When we observe his reflex motor behaviour we find that the *neck righting reflex* is still present and very strong. When the child's head is turned to the right his body will immediately begin to turn in the same direction. The *Moro Reflex* is also still strong and the baby will still react to a movement of the supporting surface, or to a startling noise by a sudden abduction and extension of the arms and legs followed by a return to their normal position of adduction and flexion. *The assymmetrical tonic neck reflex* is constant with some children, but with others it only appears occasionally. It is likely to be constant and strong in the cerebral palsied baby. When it is present, the baby lies with his head turned to one side, usually the right, in a kind of fencing position, that is, with his right arm extended and his left arm flexed towards the shoulder. If a baby shows a left hand dominance his head will be turned to the left, and his left arm extended and his right flexed. As Gesell (27) notes, this behaviour channelizes the baby's vision towards the outstretched hand.

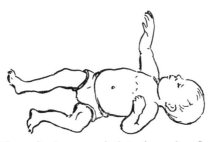

Figure 7. Assymmetrical tonic neck reflex.

The *labyrinthine righting reflex* which serves to keep the head in the normal position in space, and enables the baby to lift his head, is just beginning to make its appearance at one month. In the prone position the infant is able to lift his head for a few seconds at a time, but the movement is very weak and jerky. The reflex is absent in the supine position at this age.

THE BABY AT TWO MONTHS

His facial expression has changed during the last few weeks and is now alert. If his mother smiles at him, and catches his eye, he smiles back, and may even produce a sound that is almost akin to laughter. Greene (34) notes that "a very forward baby as early as two months will reply with coos and squeals if you encourage him with smiling and talking. Incredible as it may seem, he is already replying when addressed." The vowel sounds most frequently heard in this talking are the sounds of "a" as in "hat," "i" as in "hit," "ee" as in "he," "e" as in "bed," and "u" as in "but." In addition the consonant sounds of "h," "k," "g" and "l" may be heard, produced by chance movements of the tongue and soft palate often occurring after feeding. The infant also smacks his lips after feeding, and so occasionally produces a weak "p" or "b" sound. If he is given a rattle at this age he retains it briefly but without looking at it. His eyes are more mobile, but according to Gesell (27) they may seek distant light areas and ignore stimuli in the near field of vision.

His Reflex Behaviour

The reflex behaviour at this stage is still very predominant. The *neck righting reflex* is still continuing and is very strong. The *Moro* reflex now shows itself chiefly as a reaction to a sudden and unexpected change in the position of the body. It is not as easily elicited as before. The *labyrinthine righting reflex,* which was only faintly apparent at one month of age, is now present and distinct. The baby is able to lift up his head in a prone position, although he is not yet able to do this in a supine position.

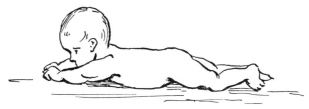

Figure 8. Labyrinthine righting reflex in a prone position.

THE RIGHTING REFLEXES AND THE CEREBRAL PALSIED INFANT

It will help us to understand the motor behaviour of the cerebral palsied infant better if at this point we examine the righting reflexes a little more closely. The Bobaths (9) make the following observations about these reflexes: "The righting reflexes play an important role in the development of the motor behaviour of the normal child. They make their appearance in a definite chronological order and are responsible for certain basic motor activities of the child. They are fully established at the age of eight to ten months, and are active up to the age of three to five years. From the third year onwards some of them become weaker and gradually disappear: others persist in a modified form throughout life. The righting reflexes enable the child to turn over from the supine to the side and prone positions, and vice versa. They initiate the first movements of raising the head in the prone and later on, in the supine position. They help the child to get on hands and knees and sit up. All these activities are at first automatic but are soon integrated into the child's volitional activities."

In severe cases of cerebral palsy, however, the righting reflexes are absent, for they are inhibited by stronger reflexes. For instance, in a cerebral palsied infant the neck righting reflex is inhibited by the stronger assymmetrical tonic neck reflex. This means that when the head is turned to the side, the body does not begin to turn in the same direction to enable the infant to turn onto its side. Instead, the turning of the head provokes the assymmetrical tonic neck reflex, with the result that the whole body automatically assumes the "fencing" attitude characteristic of this reflex. In the same way the labyrinthine righting reflex affecting the head is inhibited by the *tonic labyrinthine reflexes.* These latter reflexes cannot be seen in isolation as they interact closely with the tonic neck reflexes, but they govern the increase and decrease of extensor tone in all the limbs in different body positions. If the body is in a supine position they produce a marked increase of extensor tone. If it is in a prone position they produce a decrease of extensor tone and a marked increase of flexor tone. For instance, if the cerebral palsied infant lies in a supine position, he is likely to show stronger extensor spasticity with the head and shoulders flung back, and spine, hips and legs fully extended. If he is put in a prone position his body is likely to become totally flexed. This flexor tone is so strong that the baby is unable to lift his head, that is, to extend his neck. In other words, the labyrinthine righting reflex, which normally enables an infant to lift his head while in a prone position, has been inhibited by the stronger tonic labyrinthine reflexes.

However, as the Bobaths (9) observe, this only occurs in severe cases of cerebral palsy. In milder cases the neck righting reflex is present, and, as a result of it the infant is able to turn from a supine position onto his side. He may have difficulty in doing this, and he may do it in an abnormal way, but he does manage it. The labyrinthine righting reflex is also usually present in less severe cases. The baby is able to lift his head in both a prone and a supine position, although probably much later than the normal baby.

THE BABY AT THREE MONTHS

He can sit with support, hold a rattle and even glance

at it in his hand. In fact, for the first time he begins to look at his own hands, which marks a great step forward in hand-eye co-ordination. His eyes follow a moving object for a short distance. There is a marked decrease in crying and an increase in "talking" vocalization. He begins to move his tongue, lips and jaw, and some children begin to use repetitive chains of sound, such as "gagagagaga" when they are feeling well fed and content. The consonant sounds of "k" and "g" are heard more frequently.

Gesell and Ilg (29) note that at this stage there is a temptation to feed the baby solids, but they point out that this is unwise, as his neuro-muscular system is not yet mature enough to handle solid foods completely. For one thing, his tongue projection and lip constriction patterns are still so dominant that they interfere with the normal swallowing mechanism. In this connection it is interesting to note that recent research has indicated the frequent persistence of infantile swallowing, with its influence on speech. Possibly this may be the result of the early forcing of solid foods on a child who is not yet ready for them. Gesell and Ilg (29) believe that a baby is not likely to be mature enough to handle solids until he is about twenty weeks.

His Reflex Behaviour

The *neck righting reflex* is still evident, except, as we have observed, in infants with severe cerebral palsy. The *Moro reflex* is also still present, but it is weakening slightly. The baby seems to be building up some slight tolerance of disturbing outside influences so that he is not so easily startled as he was, for instance, at one month. The cerebral palsied infant, however, is still likely to show a strong "startle" reaction. The *labyrinthine righting* reflex is still developing. The baby is able to lift his head in a prone position with relative ease, but he is still unable to do this in a supine position. As we have observed, this reflex will not have developed in severe cases of cerebral palsy.

THE BABY AT FOUR MONTHS

The baby is now able to hold his head upright and enjoys sitting in a propped position. He is becoming both more perceptive and more expressive. He looks from object to object and he smiles at the mere sight of a face. Goldschmidt and Gesell (32) note that at four months he anticipates feeding with an open mouth when seeing either breast or bottle. He sucks strongly, but he can inhibit both the biting and sucking reflexes. This is shown by the fact that he will inhibit sucking while giving the nipple of his feeding bottle time to refill. This developmental stage in the normal baby's feeding habits will be of importance when we come to discuss the pre-speech activities of the cerebral palsy child. Choking still remains as a reflex and will continue until chewing is established. The baby's hand is beginning to loosen up, and he is becoming aware of his fingers, playing with them and putting them into his mouth. True babbling begins to make its first appearance at three to four months, marking an advance in the acquisition of speech skills. Van Riper (84) points out that the early "comfort sounds associated with feeding will still be appearing when the babbling stage begins." The babbling consists of repetitive strings of syllables or sounds, such as "dadadadadada," "gugugugugu," "mumumumumu," which the baby plays with, whispering, vocalizing, and changing them in a variety of ways, and usually when he is alone.

His Reflex Behaviour

At four months the *neck righting reflex* is still present, but the *Moro reflex* is continuing to weaken slightly. The *labyrinthine righting reflex* is gaining in strength. The baby is not only able to lift his head easily when he is in the prone position, but he is beginning to lift it briefly in the supine position as well. At present the movement is very weak, but as the reflex continues to gain strength during the next two months he will be able to achieve this more easily. He is now bidextrous, both arms moving in unison.

THE BABY AT FIVE MONTHS

He is close to sitting without support, and he can achieve it momentarily at this age. His eyes follow a dangling ring both to the right and to the left. Gesell (27) observes that he "takes hold of the world with his eyes long before he takes hold of it with his hands;" nevertheless, he is using his hands more. He pats a bottle. If an object is put into his hands he puts it into his mouth, but he does not yet reach out for it himself. He is mature enough now to handle solids. This calls for greater movement of his tongue and jaw which will have a bearing on his developing speech.

At five months we find a marked increase of babbling. The baby acquires variations in pitch so that his babbling begins to take on a conversational tone. It is not linked with specific objects, people or situations, but is simply a form of playful activity, giving the baby a wonderful opportunity to learn to control the different muscles connected with the speech mechanism. Van Riper (84) describes the importance of a baby's babbling in the following way: "He needs this vocal play to practice repeatedly all the sounds used in English or any other language. Babbling is so vitally important in the learning of talking that adults with defective speech are sometimes taught to do it by the hour." We will need to remember this when later on we discuss ways in which we can help the cerebral palsied child to acquire speech.

Irwin (47), in his analysis of the non-crying sounds of older babies shows that, by the end of the fourth month, front vowel sounds constitute only 57 per cent of the vowels heard, as against 92 per cent produced by the newborn infant. The middle vowel sounds have increased from 7 per cent to 26 per cent, and back vowel sounds from 1 per cent to 16 per cent. The analysis of consonant sounds demonstrates that during the second quarter of the first year the glottal "h" constitutes 60 per cent of all consonants heard. The sound of "g" is used about 20 per cent of the time: "m," "n," "v," "d," "w," "l" constitute about 10 per cent, and the sounds "t," "f," "v," and "z" amount to less than 1 per cent.

His Reflex Behaviour

The neck righting reflex is still present and strong. *The Moro reflex* is continuing to weaken, while the *labyrinthine righting reflex* is increasing in strength. It is now easier for the baby to lift his head when lying in a supine position than it was at four months. In another month he will be able to lift it almost as easily in this position as he can in the prone position.

THE BABY AT SIX MONTHS

When lying in a supine position, he can lift his buttocks and support himself on his shoulders and feet. In this way he extends his spine and hips, and so prepares himself for sitting, standing and walking. He can get onto his hands and knees—an accomplishment that a cerebral palsied child is not likely to achieve for a very long time. If he is given a rattle, he now retains it. He grasps a cube with his whole hand, and in pronation, that is, with the palm facing downwards. His eyes and hands are more closely coordinated, and he looks at what he is doing with his hands. This represents a more advanced behaviour pattern. The babbling increases, and he begins to use gesture and expression as a means of communication. He also begins to understand the gestures of others.

His Reflex Behaviour

The neck righting reflex is still present and strong, and the *Moro reflex* is still continuing to disappear. The *labyrinthine righting reflex* is still increasing in strength, and the baby is now able to lift up his head as easily in the supine as in the prone position.

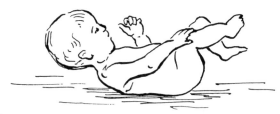

Figure 9. Labyrinthine righting reflex in a supine position.

At this time the *Landau reflex* makes a first weak appearance. The Landau reflex consists of an extension of the head, spine and legs if the baby is held free in the air, but supported under the abdomen. If the head is passively flexed in this position the whole body flexes.

The Bobaths (9) make the observation that in most children with cerebral palsy the Landau reflex is not present. They are not able to lift the head in this position, due to the inhibition of the

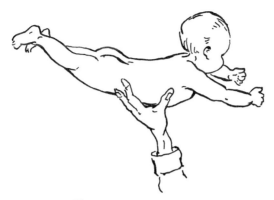

Figure 10. Landau reflex.

labyrinthine righting reflex by the tonic labyrinthine reflexes. It will be remembered that we have already discussed the way in which these latter reflexes prevented the cerebral palsied child from lifting his head when lying in a prone position at an earlier stage of his motor development. Now at six months these same reflexes are preventing him from lifting his head when held free in the air in a prone position.

At six months we also find another new reflex, the *protective extension* of the arms. According to the Bobaths (9) this reaction appears at this age and remains throughout life. It consists of an extension of the arms and hands as a protection from injury in falling. In children with cerebral palsy whose upper extremities are affected, the reaction is absent. This is why they need helmets.

THE BABY AT SEVEN MONTHS

At this age the baby transfers objects from hand to hand, sucks and bites them, and then takes them away and looks at them. Gesell and Ilg (29) have made the point that the baby's throat muscles are much more highly organized than they were at four months, and that as a result, he can now "handle" solids with ease. When being fed he can use his lips and tongue with greater precision, and he closes his mouth firmly when he has had enough. He is beginning to cut his first teeth. Goldschmidt and Gesell (32) observe the first signs of chewing at this age, the baby using his tongue to transfer lumps of food around his mouth. As the chewing develops, so the choking reflex becomes inhibited, denoting a great advance in the neuro-muscular organization of the child. This stage will be of importance when we come to discuss the prespeech activities of the cerebral palsied child. We also hear a much wider variety in his babbling. At times, he practices combinations of sounds for several days. Van Riper (83) gives the following account of this behaviour: "During the last quarter of the first year the baby often plays with a certain sound or syllable for days at a time, repeating it over and over again until the parent feels like changing the record. But this is his practice period—his dress rehearsal for talking."

His Reflex Behaviour

At seven months we see the first appearance of the *body righting reflex acting on the body*. This reflex, as the Bobaths (9) point out, plays an important role in the child's early attempts at getting up, sitting and standing, and it also modifies the neck righting reflex. For example, whereas in the first six months of life the turning of the head to one side is followed by the turning of the whole body, the development of the body righting reflex at about seven months confines this movement to a rotation of the body between the shoulders and the pelvis. (Thus a more refined movement pattern develops out of and supersedes an earlier and more primitive one.) In describing the role of the body righting reflex in sitting, the Bobaths (9) write: "Up to the age of fourteen months most children, if not allowed to pull themselves up with their hands, sit up by first turning over on their abdomen, then by getting on hands and knees, and finally, by sitting up or getting on their feet. This rotation around the body axis gradually decreases until, towards the age of three years, children sit up with only slight rotation, using one hand on one side to support themselves. They no longer get on hands and knees." These reflexes are nearly always absent in severe cases of cerebral palsy. Such children are unable to turn over and to sit by themselves. Milder cases learn to sit up by pulling themselves up by their arms and hands, but without any of the normal rotation of the body.

At seven months the *Moro reflex* is continuing to disappear as the child begins to build up a resistance against sudden noises and unexpected movements. The *labyrinthine righting reflex* continues to gain in strength. The *Landau* reflex, the extension of the whole body if the baby is supported under the abdomen and held free in the air, is stronger than it was a month ago. The Bobaths believe that the absence of the Landau reflex in children with cerebral palsy is a sign that they will be unable to maintain a normal upright position in standing and walking. The *protective extension of the arms,* a reflex movement to safeguard against falling, which made its first appearance at six months, is continuing to develop. This reflex remains with us all our lives and often saves us from hurting ourselves when we fall.

THE BABY AT EIGHT, NINE, AND TEN MONTHS

At eight months of age the child is able to sit without support for one minute. He is erect, but distinctly unsteady. At nine months he can sit without support for ten minutes. He can lean forward from this position, and then pull himself back into an upright position once again. A month later he can sustain a sitting position with good control, steady and erect.

At eight months a normal baby can turn by himself on to his abdomen, and with help he can stand erect. At nine months he can stand when holding on to the rail of his crib or play-pen. A month later he can pull himself to his feet, stand holding to the rail, and then lower himself again. He attempts to crawl at eight months, but has difficulty in controlling his legs. A month later he may crawl backwards, as his legs still lag if he tries to go forward. This is rectified a month later and he begins to crawl properly.

A cerebral palsied child, on the other hand, is not likely to be sitting up at eight, nine or ten months, and when he does, as we have seen, it will be in an abnormal way. If at this age an attempt is made to put such a child on to his feet, he will throw back his head, extend his whole body and stand on his toes.

Evidence seems to point to the fact that the first comprehension of true words dates from approximately the age of eight months, that is, a couple of months before the child begins to utter them himself. He is still babbling, but Van Riper (82) notes that toward the end of the eighth month inflections are beginning to appear, making the babbling resemble adult speech more closely. Also, for the first time, the child begins to imitate the adult's physical rhythmic movements, such as clapping and nodding. A month later he shows greater discrimination and comprehension of true words. For instance, the word "eat" now sets his mouth in motion. Imitation which had first appeared about the second month in connection with play, is now more exact and complex, and paves the way for the production of true words. Greene (34) makes the point that a child "is able to imitate far more easily the sounds made by his parents as long as these are in his babble vocabulary." At ten months Gesell and Ilg (29) describe the child as being more discriminating, and more perceptive of small variations in sight and sound. His increased perception makes him more sensitive to external events taking place in his environment, and so more responsive to demonstration and teaching. He makes conscious efforts to imitate. At this age he may produce his first word, which represents a whole sentence to him. If he does not produce a real word he will play with certain sounds or syllables for days at a time. Goldschmidt and Gesell (32) note that at ten months he responds to hearing his own name, and when he sees himself in a mirror he leans forward, smiles and vocalizes. His manual dexterity is also developing rapidly. At ten months not only can he grasp objects, but he is also beginning to release them. His index finger is coming into play at this time, and he uses it for poking objects and exploring inside them. This finger and his thumb are coming increasingly into opposition.

His Reflex Behaviour

The righting reflexes reach their maximal strength around the tenth month. The Bobaths (9) have observed that at this age the child is often unable to remain lying in either a supine or a prone position for any length of time. If he is placed on his back he will immediately sit up, and if he is placed on his abdomen he will immediately get onto his hands and knees. In other words, during this stage the child is unable to inhibit his righting reflexes for any length of time. The *neck righting reflex* is continuing to be modified by the *body righting reflex,* which, in turn, is increasing in strength. The *Moro reflex* is continuing to disappear, and soon all that will be left of it will be the modified "startle" reaction that will remain throughout life. In children with cerebral palsy, this reflex may still be present in its earlier and more pronounced form for many years. The *labyrinthine righting reflex* and the *Landau reflex* both reach their maximal strength during the tenth month. The *body righting reflex* and the *protective extension of the arms* are both continuing to develop.

THE BABY AT ONE YEAR

His one idea is to get on to his feet. He holds on to the rail of his crib or play pen, pulls himself up, and then takes steps first to one side and then to the other. If his hand is held he sometimes is able to walk. On his own outside the playpen, he crawls. Gesell and Ilg (29) believe that at one year the baby is in the midstream of developmental changes which will not reach fulfillment until he is fifteen months old. He now grasps objects with his finger tips, instead of with his whole hand as he did at six months, and his forefinger and thumb are now held in opposition to one another. His powers of release are maturing and he enjoys picking up and dropping objects.

Children with cerebral palsy may never develop this fine coordination between thumb and forefinger. When they grasp, if they are able to at this age, it is still likely to be with the whole hand, and their ability to release objects will not develop until later. Sometimes with serious cases it does not develop normally, and the only way these children can grasp and release is by making use of the assymmetrical tonic neck reflex. For instance, if such a child wants to pick up a block that is lying to his right, and at a little distance from him, he will turn his head to the right, which will cause his right arm, hand and fingers to extend (and rest on the block) , while his left arm flexes. In this position he is unable to flex his fingers and arm in order to pick up the block. The only way he can do this is by turning his head to the left, which will cause his left arm to extend and his right arm, hand and fingers to flex and so pick up the block. Conversely, if he wants to release the block he is unable to extend the fingers of his right hand in this position. The only way he can do this is by again turning his head to the right, which again will produce an extension of the right arm, hand and fingers, and so enable him to release the block. A child who is only able to grasp and release objects in this way can never develop the hand-eye coordination of the normal child for, as often as not, his head has to be turned away from his hands.

The one year infant chews and swallows with greater ease and with less spilling from the mouth. If he learns to walk before the first word appears, the words are usually delayed until he walks with ease. In most children, speech comes first. In their research on the development of speech Darley and Winitz (17) found that the earliest age at which normal children produce their first words is nine to ten months, and the latest age is eighteen to nineteen months. They note that the intelligence of the child seems to be an important factor in the appearance of the first word. There seems little doubt that the period between one year and thirty months is the most favourable for the development of speech. Van Riper (82) has made the point that at thirty months this favourable period is usually over, so that subsequently speech develops more slowly and with less facility than when it is begun earlier.

Cerebral palsied chlidren are usually considerably retarded in uttering their first word. In their research on this subject Denhoff and Holden (19) report a mean age of 27.1 months for the appearance of the first single words. Hood and Perlstein (42) studying a group of 179 spastic hemiplegic subjects found a mean age of 21.3 months, and with thirty subjects with I. Q.'s below 65, they found a mean age of 32.2 months. Byrne (12) however, studying a group of cerebral palsied children with normal mentality and hearing ability, found a median age of fifteen months for the appearance of the first words. Children with a hearing loss will obviously be later in producing their first word than children with normal hearing. If these children also have cerebral palsy then they will be even later still in saying their first words. Morley (60) reports that of 110 cerebral palsied children with a hearing loss, twenty-nine did not say any words. The remaining children produced their first words at four years.

Reflex Behaviour at One Year

At the time of the baby's first birthday, the *asymmetrical tonic neck reflex* has disappeared. He no longer assumes the "fencing" attitude when his head is turned to one side. However, as we have seen, this reflex is still likely to be present in cerebral palsied children, and it may become even stronger as the spasticity increases. The *neck righting reflex* is becoming weak and is not observed in many children. It is modified both by the body righting reflex and by the child's developing volitional behaviour. If he turns his head to one side when lying in a supine position he can inhibit his body from turning automatically in the same direction if he does not want to lie on his side. The *Landau reflex* is still present and the *body righting reflex* is increasing in strength at this age. It enables the baby when lying in a supine position to turn over onto his abdomen, get onto his hands and knees, sit, and then stand up. *The protective extension of the arms* is continuing to develop. As the child sits, stands and begins to walk he will need this reflex to protect himself from falling. It is still absent in cerebral palsied children.

THE CHILD AT FIFTEEN MONTHS

Patterns of behaviour that were in the making at one year have now come to fulfilment. According to Gesell and Ilg (29), the child's gross motor drive is very strong at this point. He is ceaselessly active, and beginning to insist on doing things for himself. Now that his ability to release his grasp is better developed, he delights in throwing his toys out of his baby carriage and pen. He shows and offers toys to others, often only to retrieve them again. He is discarding his nursing bottle and endeavouring to feed himself with a spoon, though sloppily. He often misses his mouth with this tool, although he can find it easily with his fingers. Cerebral palsied children, however, would have difficulty in even finding their mouths with their fingers, for this calls for a hand-eye-mouth coordination that is usually beyond their powers at this age. This coordination may develop later with milder cases, but may never develop in severe cases. As we have already observed, these latter cases may still have their motor behaviour largely dominated by the assymmetrical tonic neck reflex, which would cause them to turn their heads away as their hands approach the mouth.

Between one year and fifteen months the normal baby's comprehension of words increases steadily, but his vocabulary and use of words grow at a much slower pace. This is probably due to the fact that during this period locomotion is his chief interest. By means of crawling, propelling himself on his bottom, and walking a few shaky steps he succeeds in getting himself from one place to another. This new and exciting occupation absorbs him to the exclusion of everything else. Cerebral palsy children are unlikely to be crawling, let alone walking, at this age. As we have already described, those in whom the Landau reflex did not develop may never be able to maintain an upright position in standing and walking. Some may not even be sitting up.

We have already discussed the fact that normal children can produce their first words any time between nine or ten months and eighteen months. Therefore, the number of words that a normal child will be saying at fifteen months depends entirely on what age he produced his first words during this time span.

His Reflex Behaviour

At fifteen months the reflex picture is very much the same as it was at one year. The *neck righting reflex* is continuing to weaken, and the *Landau reflex*, according to the Bobaths (9) is present in twelve out of thirteen children. The *body righting reflex* is still active, and at this stage it is one of the factors that enables some children to make a change in their method of getting up from the supine to a sitting position, and so on to their feet. These children, by rotating their bodies, are able to get onto their hands and knees from a supine position without having first to turn over onto their abdomen. This method of getting up is a transitional stage between the earlier and more primitive one, and the later adult method of getting up symmetrically, which will not be acquired until approximately five years of age.

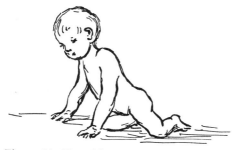

Figure 11. Transitional stage of getting up.

THE EIGHTEEN-MONTH-OLD CHILD

At this age Gesell and Ilg (29) observe that the child's motor drive is so strong that he is constantly running, going up and down stairs, constantly introducing variations into his movements. The gross motor activity takes the lead over the fine, but he can now take off his shoes, hat and mittens—skills that a cerebral palsied child will not acquire until very much later. The normal child usually has about ten words at his disposal at this age, but he needs many more to express his needs and his growing interest in his world. In the area of language his motor drive expresses itself in a flood of jargon, which is as near an imitation as he can achieve of the adult speech he hears around him. Goldschmidt and Gesell (32) observe that his ability to look at pictures and to point and name objects in them shows his growing ability to master symbols. At eighteen months his reflex behaviour is still much the same as it was at fifteen months. As his central nervous system matures his motor behaviour becomes less automatic, and more under his own voluntary control. In cerebral palsied children, however, reflex behaviour is still likely to be the more dominant.

THE TWO-YEAR-OLD CHILD

He is still geared to gross motor activity, but his fine motor control has advanced and he has better coordination than at eighteen months. He can kick a ball, and manipulate tools, first with one hand and then with the other. At two years he begins to get a little control over his organs of speech, the muscles of the jaw coming under his voluntary control. Chewing is becoming more rotary, and is not as effortful as it was at eighteen months. At two years the child cuts his last milk teeth. Jargon is disappearing, to reappear only in moments of stress, and three word sentences are coming in. The child soliloquizes when he is alone, verbalizing his immediate experiences. Goldschmidt and Gesell (32) observe that at this age the child is able to differentiate himself from his environment. He uses "I," "me" and "you," and has a vocabulary varying from about fifty to a couple of hundred words. The first half of the third year is the period during which he will acquire many new words. Imitation will be at its height between his second and third birthdays. Van Riper (84) points out that the vocal aspect of this is the development of "echolalia," a queer, dream-like repetition of words heard but not understood. Echolalia reaches its peak at thirty months, and has usually disappeared by the time the child is three.

His Reflex Behaviour

Between two and three years of age volitional activity continues to increase while reflex activity continues to decrease. According to the Bobaths (9) the *neck righting reflex* is present in only eleven out of nineteen children. The *Landau* reflex has disappeared, while the *protective extension of the arms* is increasingly present. The *body righting reflex* is enabling 50 per cent of children to get up in the transitional form already described. The remaining 50 per cent are still using the primitive method of turning over onto the abdomen and getting on the hands and knees as a preparation for sitting and standing. Cerebral palsy children are still likely to be under the domination of reflex behaviour, the more severe cases still being subject to the early and primitive assymmetrical tonic neck reflex. This reflex, as we have observed, prevents the development of the neck righting reflex which would enable the child to turn onto his side.

THE THIRTY-MONTH-OLD CHILD

He is again in a transitional period. At this age it is hard for him to modify and control both his physical and psychological behaviour. This seems largely due to the inhibitory powers of the central nervous system not yet being sufficiently developed. Physically, his flexor and extensor muscles are not yet co-ordinated in a balanced check and counter check, with the result that his grasp is too strong and his release over-violent. Psychologically, this inability to inhibit shows itself in temper tantrums and extremes of behaviour. It is as if the child is constantly being pulled into two opposite directions at once.

This period of development is likely to be a particularly painful one for the cerebral palsied child, for owing to his brain damage he lacks the ability to inhibit and control his motor behaviour. The power to inhibit which will develop of itself in the normal child, will not do so in the cerebral palsied child. Instead, he must be trained to inhibit earlier patterns of behaviour in order that more mature patterns may develop. At this stage in his development, particularly, he stands in great need of therapy along the lines we are discussing.

Most children between their second and third birthdays show a great vocabulary increase, and begin to put two short sentences together to make compound ones. However, under emotional stress they are likely to lapse back into jargon. Echolalia has reached its peak with most children, and will gradually disappear during the next six months. During this period the child begins to realize that words are made up of a series of sounds, and begins to develop the ability to discriminate between them. As a result of this he is able to correct many of his previous articulatory errors.

THE THREE-YEAR-OLD CHILD

The conflicting extremes of the two-and-a-half year old's behaviour has given way to a high degree of self-control in the three year old. Gesell and Ilg (29) believe that this self-control has a motor basis in that the child's whole motor set is more evenly balanced and fluid. His fine motor coordinations have developed, and he is able to undo his buttons and to crayon, even imitating a cross, with greater precision. He uses simple sentences with ease and many compound ones. He listens carefully to words, and practises them on his own in dramatic monologues, referring to himself by using a pronoun. Goldschmidt and Gesell (32) note that at this age the child is beginning to dissociate the spoken word from the appropriate gesture that previously had accompanied it, which marks an important advance in his linguistic ability. He will still probably have inconsistent articulatory errors in his speech which may remain until he is six or seven years old.

His Reflex Behaviour

At three years of age and onwards the child's reflex behaviour is increasingly modified by his developing cortical control, and so become increasingly voluntary. However, in this connection the Bobaths point out: "In every one of our voluntary movements is an automatic element outside our consciousness. We initiate a movement, but leave the details of its execution mainly to lower centres of integration with their automatic patterns of movement and postural adjustment."

When we come to observe the reflexes that had dominated his earlier motor behaviour, we find that traces of the *neck righting reflex* may be produced at the first examination of the child, but after that it is inhibited by him. The *protective extension of the arms* is continuing to develop, and can be seen in action protecting the child from falling. The *body righting reflex* is still active, but is gradually decreasing in strength. At three years of age a normal child can sit up by using one hand for support and with only a slight rotation of the body. At five years of age this righting reflex will be inhibited and the child will get up like an adult.

Looking back over this brief description of the motor behaviour of the normal child we cannot but be impressed by the orderly way in which it evolves. Step by step we see specific activities developing out of the more general activities that preceded them. We see more mature movement patterns superseding the earlier and more primitive reflex activities. This progression of motor behaviour from the more primitive to the more mature is, of course, brought about by the slow maturation of the central nervous system. As higher centres of the brain slowly develop the normal infant's motor behaviour changes in step with this process. In children with cerebral palsy this orderly progression does not take place. Owing to the brain damage, the central nervous system does not mature of itself, with the result that motor behaviour often remains at a primitive reflex level.

Chapter V

ASSESSING THE PROBLEM

WE have discussed the neurological and speech development of the normal child at some length because it gives the necessary background for the treatment of the cerebral palsied child. In treating him it is essential at all stages to measure his performance against that of the normal child, and to follow the normal developmental pattern as closely as possible. If a cerebral palsied child is able to start speech therapy before he has begun to talk, then his speech development is more likely to follow that of the normal child, but, of course, at a much slower pace. However, if he starts therapy after he has already begun to talk, but in an abnormal way, then the therapist needs to be able to measure his performance against that of the normal child in order to find out which of the earlier skills, or prerequisites for speech he has, or has not, mastered. As in his physical therapy the cerebral palsied child needs to be helped to master the earlier skills so far as he is able, in order to prepare the way for the development of the more mature and intricate speech skills.

THE SPEECH ASSESSMENT

The most effective way of measuring the cerebral palsied child's performance seems to be by making a detailed speech assessment covering four main areas. First, an assessment should be made of his ability to move those parts of his body associated with his speech mechanisms, such as his head, neck and shoulders. Secondly, an evaluation should be made of such vegetative activities as sucking, swallowing, biting and chewing, for these are prerequisites for speech, and also of his breathing. Thirdly, an assessment should be made of his ability to move and manipulate his organs of speech, such as the jaw, lips and tongue. Fourthly, his ability to vocalize and speak must be evaluated.

In making this speech assessment, it is necessary to find out which of the patient's reactions are normal, which are pathological, and which are primitive but normal. Again, with each reaction tested it is necessary to find out which movement the patient is able to do voluntarily, both with and without emotional stimulation, and which he can only do involuntarily, or merely as a reflex movement in response to a stimulus. This assessment, as we have already indicated, needs to be carried out before the commencement of treatment, and also periodically throughout the treatment in order to check if any changes have taken place.

Following the normal neurological development the speech assessment starts with the more gross and primitive movements and works towards the finer and more mature movements. It is usually carried out with the patient lying on a plinth, or cot, in a reflex inhibiting posture to which he has become accustomed in his physical therapy. Such a posture could be a supine one, but with the legs hanging over the edge of the plinth (in order to break up the pattern of total extension), and the arms extended by the sides.

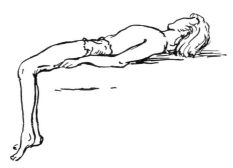

Figure 12. Supine reflex inhibiting posture with knees flexed over end of plinth.

An easier position for a more handicapped patient would be a side-lying position, either with the head flexed forward or not, as required by the individual patient (see Fig. 6).

Head and Shoulder Movements

We usually begin our assessment with the observation of the patient's head and shoulder movements, in order to see how well he can dissociate the one from the other. Starting with the shoulder movements, we first see if the patient can allow a passive upward movement of one shoulder (as in shrugging the shoulders) without an associated movement of the other. This needs to be tried out on both the right and left shoulders. If he can do this, we then see if he can carry out the same procedure voluntarily.

Our next step is to find out whether the patient's head can move without an associated movement of the shoulders. First, we turn his head passively to the right, and then to the left, and observe whether the shoulders or the rest of the body rotate in the same direction. In less severe cases we may find that the body will follow the head, showing the influence of the neck righting reflex, which, as we have already seen, is a primitive but normal reflex. Such cases, in accordance with the normal developmental pattern, are likely to be ready for speech therapy. If the turning of the head produces the assymmetrical tonic neck reflex, as may happen with severe cases, this is usually a sign that the patient is not yet ready for speech therapy, for his abnormal reflex patterns of movement have not yet been sufficiently inhibited. With milder cases we can see if the patient is able to turn his head voluntarily, first, to the right, and then to the left.

Another way of testing the dissociation of the movements of the head from the movements of the shoulders is to flex the patient's shoulders forward (as he lies in a supine position) and see if his head will fall back. If it does then this is an indication that his abnormal reflex patterns of total flexion or extension have been broken up, in that he is now able to flex his shoulders while extending his neck. The patient whose head flexes forward when his shoulders are flexed, shows that he is still under the influence of primitive reflex activity, and he probably will not be ready for speech therapy.

Another indication of whether the patient's abnormal reflex patterns have been inhibited is if he can raise his head when lying in a prone position. As we have seen, it is the action of the labyrinthine righting reflex which enables the normal baby to achieve this at two months of age. If the cerebral palsied child can do it when he is being assessed for speech therapy, it means that his primitive but normal reflex is beginning to operate. The ability to raise his head when lying in a supine position is not fully developed in the normal baby until he is six months of age, so that it may not yet have developed in the cerebral palsied child, but we should check to see.

We also need to observe whether the assymmetrical tonic neck reflex is present when the child's head is turned either to the right or to the left. In normal children, as we know, this reflex is sometimes still apparent up to the age of four months, but it is more usual for it to have disappeared by about six weeks of age, or a little later. With severely handicapped cerebral palsied children it sometimes gets stronger and more pronounced as they get older. The cerebral palsied child who is still under the influence of this reflex is also not likely to be ready for speech therapy.

Having tested the patient's ability to turn his head voluntarily to both the right and the left, we need to find out if we can turn it passively in either direction. This will give us an indication of the state of his muscle tone. If we have difficulty in turning it, there is every likelihood that his muscle tone is abnormally high; and if it turns almost too easily, and the muscles of the neck seem very floppy, it is probably abnormally low. An athetoid, of course, will fluctuate between high and low muscle tone.

Laughing, Crying and Coughing

Having assessed the patient's head and shoulder movements, we next consider activities that are more closely related to speech, such as laughing, crying and coughing. In all these activities the child is using his voice, and conscious vocalization is often one of the main stumbling blocks for the cerebral palsied patient. Therefore, the way in which he vocalizes in these related activities may well throw a light on his ability to vocalize for speech.

Laughing, being associated with a pleasant, relaxed feeling, is probably the easiest of these activities, and gives a better indication of the child's normal voice than, for instance, crying. The child who laughs spontaneously and normally is likely to find it relatively easy to vocalize for speech. The child who laughs silently, or whose laughter is accompanied by associated body movements and facial grimaces may have greater difficulty.

Abnormal crying is related to abnormal vocalization in the same way. For example, a child who holds his breath when he is crying is likely to do the same when he attempts to speak. A child who screams rather than cries is also likely to find it difficult to produce voice without a great deal of tension and forcing. A child who has a lot of phlegm and easily becomes choked when crying will probably have the same difficulty when he starts to speak. On the other hand, the prognosis is good for the child who cries normally.

Coughing is another yardstick. A great many cerebral palsied patients have great difficulty in coughing, probably because it is often initially, more of a voluntary, than an involuntary, act, and any voluntary behaviour is difficult for such a patient. Also, a great many have an undue amount of mucus and phlegm which increases the difficulty of initiating a cough to clear the throat. It is as well to discover whether the individual patient has the ability to cough voluntarily, or whether he only coughs involuntary, or indeed, whether he is able to cough at all.

Sucking and Swallowing

We come now to the assessment of sucking and swallowing which are necessary activities in the development of speech. As we have already described, sucking is a reflex activity which manifests itself at birth. It is provoked by hunger, and also by any stimulation in the region of the mouth, whether it be the touch of the nipple, or some object unrelated to food. At four months the normal baby, although still sucking strongly is able to inhibit it while waiting for the nipple of his feeding bottle to refill.

When we come to evaluate the sucking of a cerebral palsied child, we need to find out whether his sucking is purely a reflex activity, as it is with the newborn infant, or whether he can suck voluntarily. We also need to know whether he is able to inhibit his sucking, even if the stimulation goes on. This has a particular significance for his speech development, since he will not develop the more mature chewing reflex until he can voluntarily inhibit the more primitive sucking reflex. If the child can suck we also need to know in what position he can suck most easily. This is likely to be in those postures which inhibit his abnormal reflex activity most effectively. This has to be verified. It is also important for us to know if such abnormal reactions as closing of the fists or eyes, or facial grimaces occur simultaneously with the sucking. The child who cannot move any parts of his speech mechanism without associated body movements or facial grimacing is likely to have the same difficulty when he attempts to speak.

There is, of course, a very close relationship between sucking and swallowing in the infant. For example, the question of whether he was breast- or bottle-fed is of importance for it may have a bearing on his swallowing habits. Straub (81) believes that abnormal swallowing habits may develop in bottle-fed babies who are given feeding bottles with the wrong kind of nipple. According to him, this nipple is a long one with several holes, and he describes the results of using it in this way: "An infant's mouth is very small, and this long nipple which fits halfway down his throat, will not let him put his tongue against the roof of his mouth, even if he wants to. He cannot suck and swallow properly for, as he sucks, the milk comes so freely that he will either regurgitate and choke or spill milk out at the sides of his mouth. In self-defence, the child puts his tongue forward and grasps the nipple between the gum pads and tongue and swallows with his tongue in this position. Children who swallow in this way from birth may go through life swallowing abnormally." We might add that they may also go through life speaking abnormally, for this tongue thrust (or "reverse" swallow as it is sometimes called) has unfortunate implications for speech. The child who thrusts his tongue forward as he swallows, may also thrust his tongue forward as he says "s," "sh," "ch," "j"; in other words, he may very well lisp. He is also likely to say tongue tip sounds, such as "t," "d," "l" and "n" with his tongue pressed forward against his incisors rather than up against the teeth or alveolar ridges.

Therefore, in examining a cerebral palsied child it is important to get an account of his early feeding habits. If he is a bottle-fed baby, not only must we observe his swallowing carefully, but we must also bear in mind that this method of early feeding may have had some repercussions in the interpersonal relationship with his mother that we have already discussed. We also need to know whether he is able to swallow voluntarily, as a normal child begins to do when he starts chewing, or whether the movement is still merely a reflex one as in the newborn.

There is also a close connection between swallowing and drooling. The cerebral palsied child who is not able to swallow voluntarily, and who also has an abnormal swallow is likely to have trouble with drooling. We need to get as much information as we can about this since drooling is often a major obstacle in the acquisition of speech.

Choking, a reflex which occurs in the newborn infant, and is not inhibited in the normal child until he begins to chew, may add to the cerebral palsied child's feeding difficulties. Even when he has begun to chew it may still remain with him for some time.

Biting and Chewing

If a newborn infant is touched in the close vicinity of the mouth (or if his gums are touched), he will respond by making a reflex biting movement, which consists of a continuous opening and closing of the jaws. In the normal baby it becomes inhibited by the development of the chewing reflex between seven and eleven months of age.

This primitive but normal reflex is very often pronounced in cerebral palsied children. If it is allowed to remain unchecked it will delay the development of the chewing reflex, and so retard the child's speech development. Therefore, in our examination of the child we need to assess the strength of this reflex, and discover the stimulus that evokes it. With some children the mere sight of a hand approaching their mouth is enough; with others it may be the touching of their incisors or gums, or the touching of their side molars and gums. We also need to discover if the child is able to inhibit this reflex activity even when the stimulation continues.

Chewing

We need to pay especial attention to the assessment of the chewing reflex, for this has important significance for speech. In the act of chewing the child is using the jaw, lips and tongue in a more mature and coordinated way than he has done before, and out of these gross movements will develop the fine movements necessary for speech. In examining the cerebral palsied child we need to establish three points. *First,* has the child reached the neuro-muscular level of development that enables him to chew? *Second,* if he is chewing, is the activity only a reflex one, or can he chew voluntarily; and *third,* can the child inhibit this activity?

The type of food the child is being given is also a question that concerns us. It sometimes happens that cerebral palsied children are given too much soft food, and not enough solids that make chewing necessary. This will retard their speech development, for a child will not attempt to use his jaw, lips and tongue for speech until he has had practice in using them in the more gross movement of chewing.

Jaw Movements and Teeth

We now suggest an examination of the individual organs of speech to determine whether they are being moved in a normal way. We usually start with jaw movements, for these are more gross than the movements of the lips and tongue. In examining a cerebral palsied child we first need to determine the habitual position of the jaw when the child is not speaking, or attempting to speak. Very often there is a deviation to the side that shows the greatest spasticity, and when the child opens his mouth to speak, this deviation is still present. Sometimes the jaw is thrust abnormally far forward, and this is often associated with the tongue thrust which, in turn, of course, is associated with an abnormal swallow.

Having verified the habitual jaw position we need to find out how easily it can be moved. Here we use passive movements before asking the child to make the movement voluntarily. With severely handicapped spastic children the jaw is often held tightly clenched, and only opens with great difficulty, and then into an over-wide position. This abnormal condition will need to be rectified during therapy, for in speech the jaw needs to move quickly and easily with small openings. With a milder case we need to ascertain whether the child can control the intermediate stages of opening and closing, which are so important in normal speech. We also need to find out whether he can open his mouth with his head flexed forward and close it with his head dropped back. The inability to do this, of course, is associated with the primitive reflex patterns of total flexion and total extension, and it is to be hoped that by the time the child comes for his speech examination that these reflex patterns will be in the process of being broken up and inhibited. Obviously the cerebral palsy child, like the normal child, must be able to open and close his mouth regardless of the position of his body.

When we come to observe the child's teeth we need to note whether he has the full set of milk (deciduous) teeth, and whether he also has some second teeth. We need to find out whether he can use the front teeth for voluntary biting, and the back teeth for voluntary chewing. Most important of all, we need to observe if he has any dental abnormalities. If he has an abnormal swallow, which causes his tongue to be habitually pressed forward between his teeth, there is every probability that he will have an abnormal bite. Straub (81) cites the case of a child whose tongue was habitually between his teeth, and was being thrust even further forward every time he swallowed (which is twice a minute during waking and once a minute during sleep). As a natural result of these abnormalities he developed an open bite, consisting of a gap between the central incisors when the posterior teeth were clenched. Straub states that orthodontic treatment would be useless as long as the child had these faulty tongue habits, for he needed the space between his front teeth for his tongue. If, however, the abnormal swallow could be corrected, then orthodontic treatment would be able to close the open bite.

The Soft Palate, Lips and Tongue

If the cerebral palsied child is able to produce voice, then probably the best way of finding out whether his soft palate is functioning at it should is to listen to the quality of that voice. If it is unduly nasal, as it often is with these children, we can be sure that the soft palate has not been raised to close off the nasal passage. Or, we can get him to make the sound of "ah," and see for ourselves how the soft palate responds. If he cannot voice, then we are unlikely to be able to observe it in action, for any attempt to inhale a short, quick breath (which in a normal child would produce a movement of the palate) would require greater control than he probably possesses at that point.

We come now to an assessment of the child's lips, and lip movements. First, we need to observe the habitual position of his lips when he is silent. Severely handicapped spastics are apt to have their lips drawn back into what has been described as the "spastic grin." This is associated particularly with extensor spasticity. The patient's whole body extends, his head is flung back, and his cheeks and lips are also drawn back. Other children may have their lips pursed forward in an abnormal way, with a strong line running down from the wing of the nose. This facial grimace is another aspect of the tongue thrust swallow. Both the tongue and the lips (and sometimes the lower jaw also) come forward every time the child swallows. It is important for us to observe the basic lip position, for it is from this position that the patient will begin to move his lips for speech. If it is an abnormal position then he will move his lips in an abnormal way. In assessing the lip movements we need to find out first, whether the child can smack his lips voluntarily (an accomplishment that the normal baby acquires as early as two months), and then whether he can purse and widen them voluntarily, or only as part of a reflex movement.

When we come to examine the child's tongue and tongue movements we should first observe the position in which it is habitually held. If when the child is not speaking we can see his tongue between his teeth, then there is every probability that he has the tongue thrust swallow. On the other hand, if it is not visible then his swallow is probably normal. To assess the mobility of the tongue we ask the child to put out his tongue, pull it in, put the tip first to one corner of his mouth, and then the other. With his lips apart we ask him to touch his top lip with tongue tip and then his lower lip; to touch up behind his top teeth, and then down behind his bottom teeth. In these movements we need to observe how pointed the child can make his tongue tip, and whether he is able to move it without associated head or body movements, and without facial grimacing. The child who moves his head as he moves his tongue will do the same when he begins to speak.

In milder cases of cerebral palsy we need to discover if the child is able to move his tongue independently of his jaw. In chewing, the lips, tongue and jaw move together in a slow and gross movement. But in speech although there is a subtle co-ordination between the three, each is required to move independently of the other. The tongue is geared to move with far greater precision and speed than the jaw, a speed that is required in normal articulation. Therefore, if a child can only move his tongue at the same speed as his jaw, his articulation will be slow and clumsy. Some normal children have this difficulty and have to be trained to move the tongue independently of the jaw. This being the case, it is not surprising that children with mild cerebral palsy should also have the same difficulty. Severe cases of cerebral palsy are unlikely to reach the level of neuro-muscular development that makes such movements possible.

Sensitivity

According to Goldschmidt (31), hypersensitivity in and around the mouth of the normal baby disappears by about the seventh or eighth month. With cerebral palsied children it lasts much longer. This is a matter of importance for the speech therapist trained in this approach to cerebral palsy. In the same way as the physical therapist inhibits and facilitates gross movements for the child, the speech therapist has to inhibit and facilitate movements of his speech mechanism. This, naturally enough, entails the manipulation of his head, neck, jaw, cheeks, chin, lips and tongue. The sensitivity of these parts then, needs to be assessed so that the therapist can plan a program of desensitization, that is, a systematic building up of the child's tolerance to the handling of these parts.

In such an evaluation of sensitivity we need to start with those parts which are furthest away from the mouth, which is the most sensitive, and work towards the mouth. First, we handle the child's head and neck, then his forehead and cheeks, his chin and lips. Then we need to go inside his mouth and touch the inside of his cheeks, his molar gums, both upper and lower on both sides; his incisor gums in the same way, and finally, his tongue. We need to observe his reaction to this handling. Some children may be so hypersensitive that they will react with a spasm even when their head and neck are touched. If this is the case, then on this first assessment we make no attempt to approach nearer to the mouth. Other children, usually milder cases, will have greater tolerance, but they all are likely to show some degree of sensitivity.

Breathing

We now need to evaluate the child's breathing patterns, for they will determine the quality of his vocalization. Normal speech requires a relatively slow breathing rate, in that having taken in a quick breath we then say a series of words before taking another inhalation. Westlake and Rutherford (87) note that the breathing rates of very young infants are extremely variable, ranging from twenty to forty inhalations and exhalations per minute. But by the time the normal child is two years old his rate should be stabilized in the low twenties. If a child of this age or older has a breathing rate of over thirty cycles per minute this is likely to interfere with the continuity of his speech.

Breathing patterns change with maturity. Very young infants usually show predominantly abdominal breathing for their ribs are horizontal, and any attempt to raise them would compress the thorax. This continues until they are approximately three years of age when, as a result of being erect and walking, the rib cage begins to slope downwards, and thoracic breathing becomes possible. Westlake and Rutherford (87) observe that "reversed breathing, a general term for depression of the upper chest during inhalation, is normal in some very young infants and disappears within the first few months of life." It very often remains as a breathing characteristic of cerebral palsied children. Van Riper and Irwin (85) make the point that in his efforts to get more air for phonation, a severe spastic will contract both his thoracic and abdominal muscles simultaneously, whereas, normally when we start to talk the thoracic muscles are relaxed and their antagonists, the abdominal muscles, are contracted. Research has shown that this breathing characteristic of cerebral palsied patients decreases when they are not talking, and all but disappears during sleep. Therefore, when we come to assess the breathing patterns of the cerebral palsied child we need to observe which part of his chest or abdomen he uses under these different conditions. We also need to observe whether in the case of a severely handicapped patient inhalation is allied to extensor spasticity, and exhalation to flexor spasticity. We have already mentioned the possibility of this alliance. In addition, we need to find out whether the child can breathe silently both when he is asleep and awake. Some cerebral palsied children are chronic "noisey" breathers, often due to the congestion of the throat and nose, or to the flapping of the soft palate, which often produces a noise like snoring, or to stridor from partially approximated vocal folds. We need to observe if the breathing is accompanied by head or body movements. If it is, then the child is likely to make the same movements when he speaks. It is also important for us to know whether he can hold his breath voluntarily, and whether he can blow. In other words, the more information we can get about his breathing, the greater understanding we shall have concerning his vocalization potential.

Vocalization

Producing a voice "on demand" may well be beyond the powers of a severely handicapped cerebral palsied patient. He may be able to vocalize when he is alone, or when he is in a familiar situation where there is no pressure whatever on him, but at first, in a clinical situation he is likely to fail. Or, as Van Riper and Irwin (85) observe, he may begin to phonate strongly but quickly "run out of breath," so that his voice dies away. If he then struggles to get more air he is likely to have muscular spasms which effectively prevent further vocalization. In this first assessment we may fail to get any voicing from the patient with a severe speech involvement. With less severe cases we can see if the child is able to sustain his tone, and also interrupt it voluntarily. We can listen to the quality of his voice, with particular regard to nasality, and we can observe whether he is able to change the pitch of his voice.

Speech

Some cerebral palsied children we examine will have no speech for us to assess. Others who can speak at home will be unable to do so in more unfamiliar surroundings, and under conditions of greater pressure. In these circumstances their only response to speech will be a spasm and a reversion to their former abnormal reflex behaviour. If they attempt to initiate speech they will also react in the same way. With milder cases we need to assess their ability to say words and sentences, and to articulate the individual vowel and consonant sounds correctly. We need to evaluate the rate and fluency of their speech and their general language ability. We need to observe if they have any perseverative phrases (often characteristic of the brain damaged person) and whether they are able to speak under conditions of emotional stimulation.

Hearing

It is, of course, of vital importance that the cerebral palsied child's hearing should be given as thorough a check as is possible, for the hearing is often affected. It is interesting to note that sometimes there is a marked connection between a cerebral palsied child's ability to hear at a certain moment and the degree of his spasticity at that particular moment. For instance, if at a particular moment he is having severe spasms accompanied by abnormal reflex activity, he will not hear as well at that moment as when his muscle tone is reduced, and the abnormal activity has been inhibited.

This then, is the type of assessment that we suggest the

speech therapist should make before starting treatment. It will give her a comprehensive picture of the patient's readiness for therapy, and indicate the level of his neuro-muscular development. If the therapist links the information she has from her assessment to the information that the physical therapist and the occupational therapist have already procured from their assessment of the patient, she will have a firm foundation on which to base her treatment.

Chapter VI

PRINCIPLES OF SPEECH THERAPY

WE have already discussed the general principles of this approach to cerebral palsy, and the way in which they are applied to the physical therapy of the patient. We would now like to discuss them from the point of view of the speech therapist.

As we have indicated, there are three main stages in the treatment. In the first stage the *patient's pathological and abnormal reflex behaviour has to be inhibited.* In physical therapy, this means the inhibition of such reflexes as the tonic neck reflexes which prevent the child from acquiring more developmentally mature reflexes, such as the ability to roll over from a supine to a prone position, to get onto his hands and knees, or to sit.

In speech therapy, this means the inhibition of abnormal or primitive reflex behaviour which is interfering with the development of the patient's speech. For example, the cerebral palsied patient with a severe speech involvement is not able to dissociate the motor behaviour of his speech mechanism from the motor behaviour of the rest of his body. Every time he speaks, or even attempts to speak, there is an increase of muscle tone throughout the whole body, which shows itself in an increase in the abnormality of his postures and movements. Patients who are less severely involved may not have this particular difficulty, but they may not yet have acquired the ability to inhibit the primitive reflex movements related to their speech mechanism. For instance, they may not be able to inhibit the sucking and biting reflexes. This would delay the development of the more mature chewing reflex, which is a prerequisite for speech. Therefore, in speech therapy, as in physical therapy, we attempt to inhibit the reflex behaviour that is blocking the next step in the child's neuromuscular development. With one child this may mean inhibiting the movements of the shoulders so that the head and neck can begin to move freely. With another, it may mean inhibiting the chewing reflex so that the tongue may begin to move independently of the jaw as it is required to do in speech. With every case it will be different, depending on the individual patient's level of neuro-muscular development, and this level will have been ascertained from the initial assessment of his motor behaviour. The principle is that treatment begins at the point at which normal motor development is blocked.

The second stage of the treatment is the *facilitation of more developmentally mature movements*. In physical therapy the patient is put into certain postures which facilitate the development of finer and more selective movements. In speech therapy the therapist facilitates the next step in the normal neuro-muscular development of speech. This could be the facilitation of the chewing reflex, or of voicing, or babbling, or the production of real words and sentences, depending again, on the individual patient.

The third stage of the treatment is the *performance of movements under the voluntary control of the patient*. In physical therapy the goal is to enable the patient to perform voluntarily and at will, as many normal, or near normal, movements as possible, dependent on the extent of the damage to the central nervous system, and on the potential functioning of the brain. In speech therapy the aim is to enable the patient to acquire as much control over his speech mechanism as is possible for him (within the limits of the damage to his central nervous system), so that he is able to speak freely and intelligibly at will. It is likely, of course, that only the milder cases of cerebral palsy will be able to achieve this final stage.

NORMALIZING MUSCLE TONE

Before we discuss these three stages in the speech therapy of the cerebral palsied patient, we need to bear in mind that in this approach the speech therapist is as much concerned with the patient's general condition as she is with the working of his speech mechanism. She knows that the one is dependent on the other. The patient will only be able to produce a normal voice and move his jaw, lips and tongue in a normal way if his general condition at that moment is as normal as possible. This condition is largely determined by his muscle tone. If the speech therapist disregards the patient's general condition and attempts to work exclusively on his speech mechanism, she is putting herself at a disadvantage, for in all probability his muscle tone will become even more abnormal. If he is a spastic it is likely to become even higher, and if he is an athetoid or ataxic, it is likely to fluctuate between being too high or too low. With this abnormal muscle tone throughout his body it would be impossible for the patient to make anything but abnormal movements of his speech mechanism.

The first task, then, of both the physical therapist and the speech therapist is to attempt to normalize the patient's muscle tone. The best way to do this is by helping him to adjust to a reflex inhibiting posture for, as we have already described, these postures have a generally normalizing effect on the patient. The speech therapist would be well advised to choose one that the child has become accustomed to in his physical therapy. Needless to say, she will only be able to help him adjust to such a posture if she has established a good psychological relationship with him. As in the treatment of any speech handicapped person the rapport that develops betwen the therapist and the patient is, in the final analysis, the determining factor, and it is as important in this approach as in any other. In fact, it may be even more important, for in this treatment the speech therapist has greater physical contact with the patient than is usually the case.

THE INHIBITION OF ABNORMAL REFLEX BEHAVIOUR

When the patient is well adjusted to a reflex inhibiting posture so that his muscle tone has become more normal, the therapist can begin work on inhibiting his pathological (or primitive but normal) reflex behaviour, as it is related to his speech mechanism.

In inhibiting these abnormal reflexes the therapist should work from gross movements, such as movements of the head, neck and shoulders towards finer movements of the jaw, lips and tongue. For example, if we have a child with a severe speech involvement, it will probably be necessary to begin work on the head and shoulders. Such a child is usually unable to make independent movements of his head without his shoulders also becoming involved. It is as if his body from the shoulders up is one solid block, no part of which can be moved without the other. As we have already mentioned, head control, that is, the ability to lift and turn the head freely and independently of the shoulders, is a prerequisite for speech. Therefore, the therapist's aim is to train the child to move his shoulders and his neck and head independently of each other. She does this by breaking up and inhibiting the mass movements of these parts and facilitating the development of more isolated and selective movements.

A good reflex inhibiting posture in which to achieve this would be to have the child lying on a plinth, or cot, in a supine position with his arms down by his side, and his hips and knees flexed. Having assured herself that the child is well adjusted to this posture, the therapist could put her arm under his dorsal spine and encourage him to let his head fall back over her arm in a loose and relaxed way. By flexing the shoulders forward

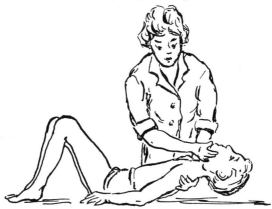

Figure 13. Supine reflex inhibiting posture with hips, knees, spine and shoulders flexed and head back.

and letting the neck extend, the therapist can break up the mass reaction of either total flexion or total extension.

Another way of breaking up this particular primitive reflex would be to have the patient also in a supine position but with his legs hanging over the end of the plinth. This time the positions of the shoulders and neck could be reversed, that is, the shoulders could be extended back and the head flexed forward.

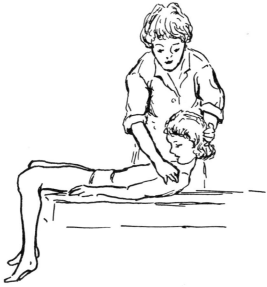

Figure 14. Supine reflex inhibiting posture with knees flexed, hips and spine extended, head flexed forward and shoulders flat on plinth.

Yet another way would be to place the child in a supine position and passively move first one shoulder and then the other, being careful to immobilize completely the one not being used. With the child in the same position, the therapist could tip the child's head first to one side (so that the ear is approached to the shoulder) and then to the other, for this will also help to dissociate the neck movements from the head movements. Holding the shoulders back and encouraging him to make small independent movements of the head also achieves the same purpose.

At first, the therapist will have to inhibit the mass reflex movement for the patient, and facilitate the smaller and more independent movements for him, but as soon as possible she should gradually abdicate her control to him. In other words, she should control and hold less, and he should control and hold more for himself. At all stages of the therapy the procedure is the same. *First,* the therapist inhibits the primitive reflexes for the patient: *second,* he begins to take over the control for himself: *third,* the therapist facilitates the new and more mature movement: and *fourth,* the patient begins to perform these movements for himself, under his own voluntary control. If at any point the therapist notices a deterioration in the patient's general condition she needs to stop and rebuild the reflex inhibiting posture again. Once such a posture has begun to deteriorate in any way it cannot be corrected, but has to be built up again from the beginning.

While carrying out this and all prespeech procedures, the therapist, naturally enough, talks to the patient to reassure and encourage him. With the intelligent older patient it is sometimes a good idea to explain the purpose of the techniques being used, provided this is done in a somewhat casual way. Too detailed an explanation is apt to increase the patient's tension.

DESENSITIZATION OF THE SPEECH MECHANISM

As soon as the speech therapist has succeeded in breaking up and inhibiting the mass movements of the patient's shoulders and head, so that he is able to move the one without the other, she needs to embark on a program of desensitization of his speech mechanism. As we mentioned before, in this approach manipulation of the patient's head, neck, jaw, cheeks, chin, lips and tongue is necessary in order to inhibit his abnormal reflex activity and to facilitate the development of more normal movements. Unless the child is systematically trained to tolerate such manipulation, he will react to it with spasms, thereby destroying his adjustment to the reflex inhibiting posture. To build up the child's tolerance, the therapist needs to hold him firmly in such a posture, and gently touch and move all the hypersensitive parts. As we described before she should start with those which are furthest away from the mouth (for this is the most sensitive part of all), and work towards the mouth.

At first the child is likely to resist, and will try to break out of the reflex inhibiting posture, and push the therapist's hands away, but this must not be allowed. The therapist needs to hold him and go on with the job, and in most cases she will find that if she goes through with this procedure regularly at the beginning of her therapy sessions, gradually the child will build up a tolerance of this handling, and allow her to touch all parts of his speech mechanism without reacting with spasms. With some children this tolerance can be built up in a matter of days, while with others it may take weeks. However long it takes, it is necessary to carry it out.

When the patient's speech mechanism has been desensitized in this way the therapist can move on to the next step in the therapy, which is to give the patient the experience of lying quietly on the plinth in a reflex inhibiting posture to which he is well adjusted, with a relaxed and quiet face free from any grimacing. For a cerebral palsied patient the first step towards acquiring normal speech is to acquire a normal face without speech. If a patient cannot lie without abnormal movements of the shoulders, head and face before attempting to speak he will certainly not be able to do so when he is attempting to speak. If the rest of the body is quiet but grimacing or facial tension still continues, the therapist must control it lightly with the tips of her fingers. As we have already described, spastic children with strong extensor spasm often have an habitual open mouth with the lips drawn back into what we call "the spastic grin." With these cases, the therapist may have to flex the head forward to inhibit the extensor spasm, and gently close the mouth for the child.

THE OPEN MOUTH AND AN ABNORMAL SWALLOW

It is important to remember, however, that there may be a connection betwen a cerebral palsied patient's chronically open mouth and an abnormal, tongue-thrust swallowing pattern. In normal swallowing the posterior teeth are brought firmly together, and as Ward, Malone, Jann and Jann (86) note the lips and cheeks remain in a relatively passive state. However, in the tongue-thrust swallow the posterior teeth are not brought together, and as Fletcher, Casteel and Bradley (26) observe, there is extreme tension in the "mouth-closing musculature" accompanied by a *forward* thrust of the tongue, causing it to protrude between the incisors. Straub (81) also refers to the typical facial grimace (the deep line running from the wing of the nose to the corner of the lips) shown by those who swallow abnormally. As swallowing takes place twice a minute during waking and once a minute during sleep, it is obvious that it has an important bearing on the mouth position of the cerebral palsied patient. If his habitual pattern is to swallow with his posterior teeth apart and his tongue thrust forward, this is likely to be his habitual mouth position, and he will find it all but impossible to keep his teeth and lips closed in what should be, a normal position.

Drooling

There is also, of course, a close connection between an abnormal swallow and drooling. As the tongue thrusts forward in the act of swallowing, the saliva is also pushed forward and out of the mouth. Drooling may occur for reasons other than an abnormal swallow. A severely involved patient may not be able to sit and hold his head up. His mouth hangs open and his tongue falls forward, causing the saliva to pour out of his mouth. A less severely involved patient with a potentially normal swallow may also have a drooling problem. This may be because he has never acquired the habit of closing his mouth, with the result that the swallow reflex has never developed as it should. Or again, drooling may be the result of a marked malocclusion of the jaw. In a study of disorders of occlusion in children with cerebral palsy, Koster (55) found that these cases showed a high incidence of malocclusion. The athetoid group were found to have the highest percentage of malocclusion with a predominantly anterior open bite. The spastic group had the next greatest percentage of malocclusion, usually with an unilateral cross-bite, while the ataxic group had varied types of malocclusion. This inability to close the teeth in a normal way reinforces the cerebral palsied patient's tendency to drool. This is particularly so with the anterior open bite of the athetoid, for in these cases, as Koster (55) observes, the saliva collects on the floor of the mouth and is pushed out by the tongue even when the patient swallows normally. If he also has a tongue-thrust swallow, drooling is likely to be a major problem.

The gradual amelioration of these manifold difficulties depends on the close cooperation between all three therapists, and, if necessary and advisable, an orthodontist. By the time the patient is ready for speech therapy he will have reached a level of neuro-muscular development when work on mouth closure can be undertaken. The correction of an abnormal tongue-thrust swallow calls for understanding and active cooperation on the part of the patient, and even with noncerebral palsied patients it is sometimes not recommended before approximately nine years of age. In the case of cerebral palsied patients it might have to be delayed even longer, but this, of course, has to be decided by the therapist in the light of the individual patient's capabilities. The basis of the treatment consists in training the patient to keep his teeth closed and his tongue tip pressed up against the alveolar ridge as he swallows, while the therapist prevents any associated movements of the lips and cheeks.

TEACHING A NORMAL MOUTH POSITION

In dealing with a patient who does not have an abnormal swallow or any serious malocclusion, the therapist's aim is to train him to acquire as normal and relaxed a mouth position as possible, for not only is this a prerequisite for the production of normal speech, but it also stimulates his swallow reflex and so helps to reduce his drooling, which all cerebral palsied patients are likely to have in some degree.

At first the therapist may have to help the child to close his teeth, in the jaw position normal for him, and then, by placing one hand gently under his chin, hold the position for him. At the same time, with her other hand, she should stroke his cheeks and lips forward, that is, against his habitual pattern, so that his whole face begins to assume a more relaxed and normal expression. Without stating her intention she should gradually release her slight pressure under his chin (but without taking her hands away) so that the patient begins to take over control for himself, and to receive the new sensations of a closed mouth. At first, he will probably only be able to hold the position for a few minutes, or even seconds, but if the therapist is ready to assume control again as soon as she perceives the necessity, these periods will gradually increase in length.

THE IMPORTANCE OF DIFFERENT BODY POSITIONS

Having achieved mouth closure successfully in one position, we suggest that the therapist should try to achieve the same thing in as many different body positions as she can, progressing from those that are easier for the child towards those which are harder for him. For example, if the child is a spastic with a strong extensor spasm the easiest position in which he could get a normal mouth position would probably be one in which the head was flexed, for the flexion of the head would help to inhibit his normal extensor spasm. The therapist, therefore, could put him into a side-lying position with his head flexed forward and work on his mouth in that position (see Fig. 6).

As soon as he has learned to keep his mouth closed normally in that, the easiest position, she should make things a little harder for him by introducing a little more extension into his posture, and yet not enough to provoke his extensor spasm. To do this, she could put him into a supine position, which extends his spine, but let his legs hang over the end of the plinth and flex his head forward (see Fig. 14).

When he can keep his mouth closed and his face relaxed in this position, she can make it a little harder for him by not flexing his head forward (see Fig. 12).

As soon as he has mastered this position, she could again make things harder for him by putting him into a position that gives him more extension. For example, she could put him on his elbows in a prone position, first, with his head flexed forward, and encourage him to let his head fall back. (See Fig. 16.)

Or, she could put him in a supine position and put her arm under his dorsal spine, so that his shoulders are flexed forward, and then held straight. (See Fig. 15.)

In this position the spastic child's reaction would be to open his mouth, but the therapist should prevent this from

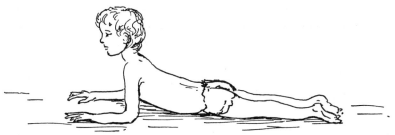

Figure 15. Prone reflex inhibiting posture with extended spine, hips and knees and flexed elbows.

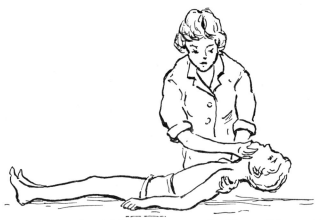

Figure 16. Supine reflex inhibiting posture with hips and knees extended, shoulders flexed and head back.

happening. In every position the procedure is exactly the same: the therapist closes the child's mouth for him: then the child takes over the control from her, first, for very short periods, and gradually for longer and longer, until finally he is able to close his mouth for himself and keep it closed under his own volition.

NEGATIVE PRACTICE

At this point, as a reinforcement of the newly acquired ability to keep a closed mouth, the well-known technique of "negative practice" could be used discreetly with some patients. In order to make the patient more aware of the difference between his old habitual open mouth and his newly closed mouth position, the therapist could ask him, first, to revert to his old habit for a short period of time, and then consciously to assume the new one. This technique highlights for the patient the difference in feeling between the two positions. If, with some patients, particularly girls, this practice is carried out in front of a mirror, the visual impression can also act as a strong reenforcement of the new ability. However, this technique has to be used with discretion by the therapist, for it calls for a degree of control that may not be possible for all patients.

THE IMPORTANCE OF SELF-CONCEPT

As soon as the patient has reached the point of being able to maintain a normal mouth position under his own voluntary control, his swallowing reflex is likely to be working more normally and, consequently, he will be drooling far less. This means that he will begin to present a more normal appearance. We believe that when this stage has been reached, the speech therapist should do her utmost to make the patient aware of this change in himself. We feel this is important because we all know from our own experience that the picture we have of ourselves has a subtle but powerful influence on our behaviour. Before receiving treatment, a cerebral palsied patient would have conceived of himself as a person continually moving (or fixed rigidly in one position) with a grimacing face and a perpetually open and drooling mouth. But now the picture has begun to change. As a result of his physical therapy the excessively abnormal postures and movements will be greatly modified, and as a result of his speech therapy the grimacing face and open, drooling mouth will have all but disappeared. The full benefit of these improvements will not be reaped until the patient is aware of them himself. If over a period of time they are brought home to him vividly enough he will gradually begin to accept them, and once he has done this at a deep enough level his concept of himself will begin to change. If he has sufficient hand control we should encourage him to explore his face (as a normal baby does) and find out for himself what it feels like so that he can get a better picture of it. If he does not have sufficient hand control on his own, then the therapist should help by moving his hands over his face. In addition, she should make full use of mirrors, snapshots, and encouraging comments from those in his immediate environment. Every imaginative effort should be made to help him to change the concept he has had of himself to one that more nearly matches his present behaviour. This may sound nebulous and unpractical, but speech therapists knowing that the successful outcome of their work often depends upon hidden causes and the underlying attitudes of the patient, will realize that this is a case in point.

THE SUCKING, SWALLOWING, BITING AND CHEWING REFLEXES

We have described the way in which the movements of the patient's shoulders can be dissociated from the movements of his head and neck so that he is able to move his head freely as he wants. As soon as a patient has developed this head control we can begin work on the finer movements of his speech mechanism, movements such as sucking, swallowing, biting and chewing.

The importance of these reflexes in the speech therapy of cerebral palsied children is now widely recognized. Palmer (67) states that the credit for the first studies on this subject should go to Muyskens (62) who, as early as 1925, was stressing the need to normalize the sucking, swallowing and chewing reflexes in cerebral palsied patients. Later research has called attention to the place of these reflexes in the normal developmental picture, and to the orderly way in which each reflex becomes inhibited in turn. For example, at four months the normal baby develops the ability to inhibit the primitive sucking and biting reflexes, although he continues to bite and suck objects voluntarily for a much longer time. The choking reflex is still present at four months, and is not in its turn inhibited until the development of the chewing reflex at approximately seven to eleven months.

THE FACILITATION OF THE SUCKING AND BITING REFLEXES

In dealing with a severely handicapped cerebral palsied child we may find that the most primitive sucking, biting and swallowing reflexes may be absent. If this is the case, then these reflexes must first be facilitated, and then, later on only, in-hibited. The touch of the nipple on the lips, or any light touch in the vicinity of the mouth, will stimulate the sucking reflex in the normal baby if he is thirsty. Westlake and Rutherford (87) note, however, that pediatric literature makes frequent mention of the fact that in many premature infants and those suspected of brain damage, tactile stimulation of the lips and inner surface of the oral cavity does not produce sucking movements. In some cerebral palsied children these sucking movements grad-ually develop, although lack of tonicity in the lips often makes the sucking weak. With others sucking does not develop. It is these cases that are of special concern to the speech therapist for, as Palmer (67) points out, developing a normal sucking (or chewing) reflex in a cerebral palsied child is a highly skilled procedure that cannot be left to the parents. A systematic pro-gram needs to be initiated by the speech therapist and carried out at home by the parents under her supervision.

We believe that the procedure developed by Palmer (67) is an effective way of teaching a cerebral palsied child to suck through a straw. In essence this consists of the following steps: (1) The parents are advised to buy a one-foot length of dental rubber tubing which has an internal diameter roughly equivalent to that of a plastic straw, and which has walls thick enough so that the tube will open again immediately when bitten. (2) When the tube has been thoroughly washed to get rid of any rubbery taste, one end is dipped into a fluid which the child particularly likes (usually either meat extracts or syrups) and about two or three inches of the tube filled with the fluid. A finger is then placed over the end of the tubing. (3) The tube is held hori-zontal and the liquid allowed to flow into the child's mouth. This procedure is carried out at regular intervals each day until the child realizes that the tube contains a liquid that he both likes and desires. With some children this may take as long as four to six weeks, but with others, considerably less. (4) As soon as the child is aware of the desirable liquid in the tube, one end of the tube is dipped in the solution and the other offered to the child. This time the tube is held slightly below the horizontal so that it will not flow. The child is then encouraged to use his lips and tongue to get the liquid. The tube is raised to the horizontal again several times and lowered again so that the child wants to work his tongue into the hole and pull it out with some of the liquid on it. This produces a weak sucking movement. The final step of this procedure is described by Palmer (67): "When a child can suck with the tube held two inches from the horizontal at the end farthest from the mouth, the tube should be brought down a little, about once a week. Each time it should be moved down from the horizontal and up from the lower position, until the child is definitely able to suck." When this pattern has been established, a straw can be substituted for the rubber tubing. The pursing of the lips around the straw, together with the liquid in the mouth will in its turn stimulate the swallowing reflex. The child should be in an easy reflex inhibiting posture as he learns to suck (such as side-lying or a supine position), and the therapist should train the parents to watch for signs of deterioration in his general physical condition. If these occur, the sucking should be stopped and the child helped to adjust to a correct posture once again.

The biting reflex can be stimulated by gently touching the child's teeth, and at the same time, with the other hand encouraging him to make rhythmic biting movements with his jaw. As the child becomes conditioned to this reflex, the stimulus can be gradually reduced until the reflex is provoked just by the sight of the hand approaching the mouth.

PSYCHOLOGICAL DESENSITIZATION

When the primitive reflexes of sucking and biting have been facilitated in these ways, the therapist needs to ensure that they can be carried out in different body positions and under varying degrees of emotional stimulation. This latter point is of particular importance. Obviously, the final goal of therapy is that the patient should be able to speak under all conditions of emotional pressure. The cerebral palsied child with his low threshold of resistance both to physical and psychological pressures will not achieve this unless the therapist systematically trains him to tolerate emotional pressures as she trained him to tolerate the physical handling of his speech organs. Without this training he will always tend to disintegrate psychologically under the pressures that are inherent in most situations and, being disintegrated, will be unable to speak.

The principle behind psychological desensitization is to put the patient under just as much emotional pressure as he can tolerate while still being able to perform an activity. Keeping a careful watch on him, the therapist should reduce the pressure just before his breaking point is reached; after a little while she should increase the pressure again, and she will find that if she reduced the pressure at the psychological moment before, this time he will be able to tolerate it a little longer. Again she should go as far as she can, and once again take off the pressure. This technique calls for a great deal of skill on the part of the therapist. Every one has his own particular way of showing tension. Some children show a barely perceptible freezing, but behind the immobility, the triggers are cocked for an explosion. Others may show a slight restlessness with a heightened colour. The therapist needs to observe the danger signals with each individual patient and be ready to remove the pressure before it becomes too much for him. If she goes too far with a cerebral palsied patient he will revert to his former abnormal reflex behaviour and the whole experience will have been lost. Handled skilfully, it can be a very useful technique in building up the patient's tolerance level.

When applying this psychological desensitization to the child who has just acquired the ability to suck and bite, the emotional stimulation could take the form of increasing disturbances in the therapy room. There could be a little more movement, a little more talking. The therapist herself could handle the child a little less carefully; her movements could be a little quicker, a little more sudden, and the tone of her voice as she speaks to him could be a little less gentle and quiet. There should be just as much emotional stimulation as the child can tolerate while still continuing to suck or bite in a normal way without extraneous movements of the rest of his body. We believe that this building up of psychological tolerance should be continued throughout the treatment so that not only does the child learn a new activity, but he also learns to perform it under varying degrees of emotional pressure.

INHIBITING THE SUCKING AND BITING REFLEXES

As soon as a child is able to suck and bite, first, as a reflex in response to a stimulus and then voluntarily and under some emotional stimulation, the time will have come for the next step in the therapy. Following the normal course of development, it will be necessary for the therapist to help the child inhibit these reflexes and facilitate the development of the more mature chewing reflex. As with a normal child the act of chewing solids will of itself help to reinforce the inhibition of the earlier and more primitive reflexes.

To inhibit the sucking reflex, the therapist again needs to have the child adjust himself to a reflex inhibiting posture, and, if possible, when he is feeling thirsty, stimulate his lips by touching them with her finger or a straw, while at the same time, with the other hand, she prevents them from moving into a sucking position. It should be mentioned here that in some children the sucking reflex is so strong that their lips begin to move into a sucking position as soon as the therapists' finger approaches their mouth. This was the case with a fourteen-year-old boy whose speech consisted mainly of jargon which he was attempting to use for communication. In spite of his age and his speech attempts, he began to suck the therapist's finger as soon as it approached his mouth. The stimuli for this reflex movement seemed to be both visual and tactual, for his lips went into a sucking position both when he saw the finger approaching his mouth and when he felt it on his lips. With this boy, and with others at the same level of neuro-muscular development this reflex needs to be inhibited so more mature mouth-behaviour can be developed. At first, the therapist will have to control the patient's lips for him by keeping them in a normal and relaxed position in spite of the stimulation. As before, the therapist should transfer this external control over to the child as soon as possible. This can be done by removing her controlling hand for a few seconds at a time, so that he experiences the stimulation on his lips and yet resists relapsing into his former reflex sucking. Gradually these moments are extended until finally he is able to inhibit the reflex for himself. Once this has been achieved, the therapist should see that the child has the same experience in different postures and under varying degrees of emotional stimulation.

At all stages of therapy it will be found that under the stress of stimulation the child will have a tendency to revert to his former immature behaviour, but in spite of this the therapist must continue systematically raising the threshold of his emotional tolerance, until he can perform the newly-acquired activity even under emotional stress.

Inhibition of the biting reflex follows exactly the same pattern. In some children this reflex is very strong, and the teeth snap together when a finger approaches the mouth, or the teeth are touched. This firm closure of the teeth prevents the development of the chewing reflex, for this calls for a measured opening and closing of the jaw. To inhibit the biting reflex the therapist must gently but firmly hold the child's mouth closed while at the same time she stimulates the reflex either by bringing her fingers close to his mouth, or by touching his teeth. Again, the same procedure of transferring the control to the child is followed.

FACILITATION OF THE CHEWING REFLEX

With the primitive sucking and biting reflexes inhibited, the speech therapist needs to turn her attention to the facilitation of the chewing reflex. This reflex, in conjunction with sucking and swallowing, is a prerequisite for speech, for it is not until a child can use his jaw, lips and tongue for these basic functions that he will be able to use them at the faster speeds required in speech. In chewing, the jaw movements are still relatively gross, although the tongue is involved in a more mature way than it is in sucking.

To facilitate the development of this reflex the speech therapist should give the child something pleasant to chew; chocolate, hard liquorice or anything else he likes, pressed laterally across the hard palate usually acts as a good stimulus. If the child is unable to move his jaws himself, the therapist should help him, and at the same time stimulate the reflex even more by rubbing his gums and teeth with her finger in a slightly rotary movement. This should be tried at the front, sides and back of both his upper and lower jaws, whichever proves the most effective. (But the therapist needs to be careful not to put her fingers in too far!) With this type of stimulation, it is hard to resist chewing, and as it develops the therapist should reduce the stimulation, so that the child gets the feeling of this movement for himself. Again the chewing should be practiced in different body positions and under carefully graded emotional stimulation. However, the best way of establishing voluntary chewing habits is by ensuring that the child is given solid food that he can chew in his daily diet. Palmer (67) makes the following recommendations to parents: "Dry sliced white bread in the oven . . . until it is *very* hard. Let the child have a piece of such bread to eat at each meal, with no butter on it and nothing to drink with it until it is all chewed and swallowed . . . He should be chewing on something most of the time. Raw carrots, potatoes, turnips, and so forth are valuable. In general, try to include in the meals, besides the bread, something that will be difficult to chew and swallow." We are in full concurrence with these suggestions and feel that it is the job of the speech therapist to orientate the occupational therapist and the parents towards putting them into effect.

The chewing of gum should also be helpful to the cerebral palsied child at this stage for it develops another skill, the voluntary inhibition of the swallowing reflex. Many cerebral palsied children unused to chewing gum will swallow it almost immediately, and they need to be trained to keep it in their mouths. This can be done by putting a piece of gum in a child's mouth, encouraging him to chew, but taking it out again in less than a minute before he has had a chance of swallowing it, or tying it to a piece of string. If this procedure is carried out once or twice a day for a period of time, the child becomes accustomed to having something in his mouth that is not swallowed. Gradually, the gum is left in for ten or twenty seconds longer, the time being increased until the child is able to keep it in his mouth and to chew for several minutes without swallowing it. Palmer (67) believes that chewing gum has a beneficial effect on the drooling problem of cerebral palsied children in that it helps to get the swallowing reflex under greater voluntary control.

SUCKING OR DRINKING

At this point in the therapy the question of whether a cerebral palsied child should suck his liquids through a straw or drink them from a cup may come up for consideration. This is of particular interest to the occupational therapist and the speech therapist for they are both concerned with the way the child manages his mouth, first for feeding, and then for speaking. However, we believe that the decision as to which the child does rests primarily with the speech therapist and should be decided in the light of the individual child's speech development. If a child is not speaking, or has very little speech we believe that he should suck all his liquids through a straw, for in the act of sucking he is strengthening muscles that he will need when he begins to speak. If he has some speech, which is not too abnormal, then we believe he could be taught to drink from a cup if he is not already doing so. In general then, the cerebral palsied child with a severe speech involvement should continue to suck his liquids through a straw until such time as he has begun to speak and has greater control over his speech organs. The milder case should be encouraged to drink from a cup. He will not, however, be able to do this in a normal way until he has learned to inhibit his sucking and biting reflexes, and this will probably not be until he has learned to chew.

JAW MOVEMENTS

When the child is able to chew gum and solids under his own voluntary control we suggest that the speech therapist should begin working on passive jaw movements in preparation for speech. The cerebral palsied patient whose speech is involved usually has great difficulty in controlling his jaw movements. He either opens his jaws too wide when he attempts to speak, or else he clenches them too tightly together, and there are none of the "in-between" stages which are so necessary in normal speaking. Children who have acquired speech before receiving treatment usually have a jaw deviation to the side that shows the greatest spasticity. This, however, is not the case with young children who have not yet begun to speak. With these children, the aim of the speech therapist should be to prevent the development of jaw deviations or abnormal jaw movements, and to produce good contact.

We believe that such a preventive program depends for its success on the habits that the child has acquired in sucking, swallowing, biting and chewing. If the therapist has been able to establish good mouth postures and movements in these activities the correct patterns will have been set, so that when the child is ready to use his jaw for speaking, he will do so in the normal way. For example, as we have already indicated, abnormal sucking and swallowing habits produce faulty tongue movements and associated jaw deviations. The therapist's aim is to prevent such abnormal movements from developing. It sometimes happens that a young child will suck and swallow normally, but begin to show jaw deviations in chewing. Great care needs to be exercised to ensure that as he chews he does not get into the habit of thrusting his jaw to one side or the other, or forward, but instead makes a normal contact in accordance with the jaw position natural for him. If this can be achieved and he has sufficient intelligence, and is not too severely involved, he will then have a good basis for acquiring speech.

However, work on the jaw is likely to be necessary with those patients who have started to speak in an abnormal way before beginning therapy. With these cases, the jaw will probably feel very stiff, and there will be great resistance to passive movements. Therefore, in first working with such a patient the therapist needs to help him to adjust to the easiest possible reflex inhibiting posture so that his general muscle tones becomes as normal as possible. Such a posture could be the side-lying one already described (see Fig. 6).

When the patient is well adjusted to this posture, the therapist can begin to move his jaw up and down. She should aim at small, fairly quick movements rather than gross ones which would be too much in accordance with his abnormal pattern of movement. Gradually, she will find that the jaw begins to loosen up. As it does so she should increase the difficulty of his posture, being careful to put him into positions in which he finds it hard either to open or close his mouth. Such positions would be with the head flexed forward (when he would have difficulty in opening his mouth), and with his head extended back (when he would have difficulty in closing his mouth). The following reflex inhibiting postures are suggested as possible ones in which passive jaw movements could be practised:

1. *Supine with flexed legs.* The patient lies with his legs hanging over the end of the plinth. The therapist puts her arm under his dorsal spine (extending it) and the patient's head falls back over her arm.

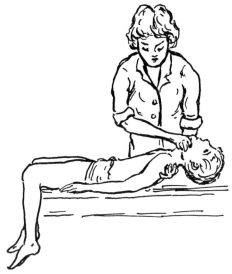

Figure 17. Supine reflex inhibiting posture with hips extended, knees and shoulders flexed and head back.

2. *Prone,* with the patient supporting himself on his elbows, and with his head held straight (see Fig. 15).

3. *Supine,* with the legs over the end of the plinth, shoulder back and head flexed forward (see Fig. 14).

4. *Sitting,* if the patient is able to sit, with the legs over the end of the plinth, the arms extended at the sides and the head held straight, tipped back, and flexed forward.

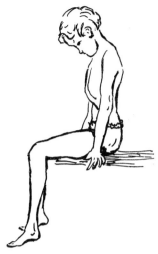

Figure 18. Sitting on end of plinth in a reflex inhibiting posture.

When the therapist is able to make small, but fairly quick, passive movements of the jaw in all these positions, she should gradually encourage the patient to begin making these movements for himself. Time and a great deal of care is necessary in making this transition from passive to active jaw movements, for the ability to move the jaw quickly and easily is one of the keys to good articulation.

THE BASIC FUNCTION OF THE ORGANS OF SPEECH

It is interesting to remember in this connection that, in speech, man is forced to use organs, muscles and groups of muscles whose basic function is to serve other purposes, namely, to suck, swallow and to chew, movements which are relatively slow and primitive in execution. In articulate speech it is necessary to manipulate these organs at a faster speed, and with far greater precision than is required of them in the performance of their basic function. Research has shown that diadochokinesis, that is the ability to perform regular, repetitive movements under conditions of speed, such as opening and closing the jaw, or raising the tongue tip, has an important bearing on the speech performance of the individual. In relating this to cerebral palsy

Heltman and Peacher (39) made a study of the rates of diadochokinesis in 102 children with spastic paralysis and found that the rates for spastics were considerably lower than those reported by Jenkins (52) for nonspastics.

At this point in the treatment then the speech therapist's aim is to help the patient to develop the finer jaw movements (necessary for speech) out of the more gross movements that were required for chewing. In chewing, the muscles of mastication bring the teeth of the two jaws together on a piece of food in a grinding movement. In speech no such firm jaw closure is made. The movement is finer and, according to Van Riper and Irwin (85) consists of a "trapdoor" movement, when the lower jaw swings "down and up like a trapdoor on an hinge," and a more subtle forward and backward sliding movement.

Not only the movements of the jaw but the movements of the tongue are also much finer and more specific in speech than they are in chewing. In sucking, swallowing and chewing the tongue moves with the jaw, whereas in speech it is necessary for it to move independently of the jaw.

DIFFICULTIES OF TONGUE DIFFERENTIATION

As soon as a cerebral palsied patient is able to move his jaw voluntarily he will have reached the stage of neuro-muscular development when it may be possible to begin work on his tongue movements.

In speech the movement of the tongue is of greater importance than the movement of the jaw, but to use it correctly calls for a degree of coordination and control that will certainly be beyond the powers of the severely involved cerebral palsied patient. A good speaker is able to move his tongue independently of his jaw and place it accurately on the precise spot in his mouth that is required for the pronunciation of any particular sound. Even noncerebral palsied individuals are sometimes unable to do this, with the result that their articulation sounds thick and clumsy. Such individuals are called "lallers," and their speech difficulty is referred to as "lalling." The main characteristic of lalling is that the finer movements of the tongue necessary for speech have not been differentiated from the grosser movement of the jaw. Thus, when the laller speaks, his tongue moves with his jaw as it does in chewing, and instead of lifting his tongue tip to make such consonant sounds as "t," "d," "l" and "n," he leaves it tucked down behind his bottom teeth and attempts to make these sounds with the blade of his tongue. The result is a thick and clumsy speech.

Naturally enough, the cerebral palsied patient will have great difficulty in dissociating the movement of his tongue from that of his jaw. As Van Riper (83) observes, he is unable to place his tongue tip accurately. "He over-shoots or under-shoots. He cannot maintain a posture. He wobbles." Owing to the damage to the central nervous system, it will be quite impossible for some cases ever to make such precise movements. If they succeed in moving their tongue with their jaws so that their speech has a lalling quality, this should be accepted and improved as far as is possible for them.

FACILITATION OF INDEPENDENT TONGUE MOVEMENTS

It may be possible for milder cases of cerebral palsy to make such tongue movements. If they have the potential, we believe that the therapist should help them by facilitating these movements for them.

The aim here is to train the patient to make an independent movement of his tongue tip up towards the alveolar ridge (behind his upper front teeth) without making an associated jaw movement. This movement is required in the correct pronunciation of such consonant sounds as "t," "d," "l," "n." To help the patient make such a movement the therapist can hold his jaws a little apart and encourage him to lift his tongue tip up and make one of these sounds by pressing it against the teeth ridge. While immobilizing the jaw in this way, the therapist has to be careful not to allow it to become "fixed." For very brief moments of time, the jaw is immobile in speech while the tongue and lips move independently of it, but on these occasions it must always be loose so that it can be mobilized again instantly.

As soon as the patient begins to make the desired tongue movement, the therapist can gradually release her hold on his jaw so that, as before in similar procedures, he begins to take over control for himself. When he is able to inhibit his jaw movement while making independent movements of his tongue, the therapist should try out this activity in different body positions and under varying degrees of emotional stimulation. This latter will be of particular importance, for much of the clarity of his articulation will depend on his ability to move his tongue freely (as is required in speech) even when under pressure.

DIFFERENTIATING LIP MOVEMENTS

Having trained the patient to move his tongue independently of his jaw, the therapist will also need to help him to dissociate the movement of his lips from that of both his jaw and his tongue. This ability is not as general as might be supposed. A number of adults and children are not able to make the "r" sound without a movement of both the tongue and the lips, and also, to a minor degree, of the jaw also. Others with a frontal lisp move their jaw, lips and tongue forward simultaneously as they pronounce the sibilant sounds of "s," "z," "sh," "ch," "j." As we have already seen, an individual with an abnormal swallow will thrust his lips, tongue and jaw forward as he swallows. This inability to dissociate the movements of his jaws, lips and tongue points to an immaturity in the development of the speech mechanism. The organs of speech are still working together as they did in their performance of their basic function of sucking, swallowing and chewing. They have failed to acquire the more mature ability to work independently of each other (and yet in a subtle coordination) as is required in speech.

If this is the case with some normal individuals it will, of course, be very general among cerebral palsied patients. It will be impossible for some, and very difficult for others. We believe that even if a patient has relatively minor brain damage it would be wiser to leave this more subtle phase of inhibition and facilitation to a later stage in the therapy.

SUMMARY

We believe that the basic principles of speech therapy in this approach to cerebral palsy are concerned with the inhibition and facilitation of successive levels of prespeech and speech behaviour. Starting at the point where normal speech development is blocked, the early vegetative activities of sucking, swallowing, biting and chewing are either inhibited or facilitated according to the needs of the individual patient. Once these activities have been facilitated by the therapist, they are practiced until the patient is able to perform them voluntarily, even under emotional stimulation. The pattern is that more immature behaviour is inhibited while more mature behaviour is facilitated at successively higher levels of the central nervous system. At the highest level the patient is trained to move his jaw, lips and tongue independently of each other. We realize, however, that only very mild cases of cerebral palsy will have the ability to make such fine and controlled movements. In more severe cases we continue to the most mature level of speech behaviour possible for the individual patient.

Chapter VII

PRODUCING VOICE

WE would now like to discuss the question of producing voice in the cerebral palsied patient. This is not too easy a problem with a child who has a severe speech involvement, for unless great care is taken he will make a great physical effort to voice, which will immediately cause a muscular spasm and a consequent reversion to his former abnormal reflex behaviour. To prevent this, we believe that voice should be produced as indirectly as possible, and only when this has been achieved should the child's attention be drawn to the fact that he is voicing.

MOVEMENT AND VOICING

We have found that the easiest and most successful way of getting voice with a cerebral palsied patient is through the use of movement. This has a sound physiological basis in that at birth, as we observed, the infant shows an instinctive urge to move as he makes noises. Every sound he makes is accompanied by a movement of his body, and this close connection between sound and movement remains with him during the first months and years of life. It is only at a later stage of development that sound and gross body movement become independent of each other.

As movement is primarily the concern of the physical therapist we believe that she can give invaluable help at this stage of the treatment. In many ways she is in a better position to get the first voicing than the speech therapist, for her attention is not focussed on getting the child to voice, but on getting him to move in a more normal way. This at once creates a more normal situation, with the emphasis in the right place. A normal baby voices spontaneously as he moves, and the more he moves the more he voices. In the same way, the cerebral palsied child stands a far better chance of voicing spontaneously if his attention is on his movements, and is not drawn to the act of phonation, as it is likely to be in the speech therapy situation. If he knows that he is required to voice then, in the early stages at least, he will immediately become tense, and this tension will interfere with the normal processes of phonation. Thus, particularly with a young child who has not yet begun to speak, the speech therapist should stand back and see if the physical therapist can, without working on it directly, encourage the child to produce voice spontaneously as he moves. If the physical therapist casually sings herself as she facilitates movements, getting the child to roll over from a supine to a prone position, or pulling him up from a supine to a sitting position, there is every chance that he will begin to vocalize too. For moving from one position to another in this way is a new and enjoyable experience for him, and quite spontaneously, he may begin to vocalize his pleasure in a normal way. This is all that some young children need. Having once discovered their own ability to voice, their speech begins to develop normally without any help from the speech therapist. With others, this spontaneous voicing is confined just to babbling, and as soon as the child begins to say real words and to use them for communication, abnormality creeps in. He begins to make efforts to speak. This immediately produces his former abnormal muscle tone and a general reversion to his reflex pattern of posture and movement. In this state he is not able to vocalize normally as he was doing at first. In view of this, we feel that when a young child begins to voice and babble spontaneously simply as a result of his physical therapy, both the physical therapist and the speech therapist must watch closely to ensure that no signs of abnormality creep in as his speech begins to develop. At the first signs of such abnormality the speech therapist should step in and begin working with the child.

THE USE OF VIBRATION

Spontaneous voicing does not always occur, particularly with severely handicapped children. In these cases, we believe that it has to be facilitated, as sucking and chewing may have been facilitated for the child.

The most effective way that we know of facilitating voice for a severely handicapped cerebral palsied child is through the use of vibration. As the child exhales, the therapist uses her spread hand to vibrate as rapidly as she can the patient's diaphragm, chest, spine, larynx, or the infrahyoid area, that is, underneath the lower jaw, depending on whichever part produces the best and quickest results. The therapist should reinforce this stimulation by producing pulses of voice herself at the same time. There are few children who can resist this form of stimulation, and if it is carried out regularly for short periods of time, at first for not more than a few minutes, it is likely to produce the desired result. The success of this technique can probably be attributed to the fact that vibration is a form of movement. The use of it to facilitate voicing helps to establish the pattern of movement and voicing shown by the normal infant. It is also effective in drawing the child's attention away from the act of phonation. His attention is drawn to the feeling of the vibration, and his voice comes as a spontaneous reaction to this.

Sometimes the physical therapist can use this technique as she works with the child, but if she is not successful in getting voice it may help if the speech therapist works with her. The physical therapist is then able to give her whole attention to normalizing the patient's muscle tone while the speech therapist vibrates one of the parts already mentioned, and vocalizes herself at the same time. Children who are severely spastic will probably find it easiest to voice when the physical therapist is facilitating movement and they find themselves free of their habitual and abnormal postures. Athetoids, on the other hand, may find it easiest when they are lying quietly on the plinth in a reflex inhibiting posture, free of their habitual movements. Both therapists need to be very relaxed and easy, drawing the child's attention away from the act of phonation as much as they are able. If he realizes that they want him to vocalize he is likely to make efforts to cooperate, which will immediately block any voicing attempts. To voice at will calls for a high degree of control which, at this stage, the child does not possess.

If the speech therapist is working on her own to produce voicing, and this may suit individual children better, we suggest that she tries the following reflex inhibiting postures.

Side-lying: here the therapist can vibrate the upper side of the ribs, the diaphragm, the larynx or the infrahyoid area (see Fig. 6).

Supine: with legs flexed unto the chest, and arms down by the sides. In this position, the therapist can vibrate the diaphragm, the lower ribs, the larynx or the infrahyoid area (see Fig. 5).

Prone: with arms stretched up above the head, and extended spine. In this position the therapist can vibrate the spine or the lower ribs.

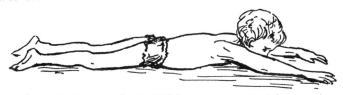

Figure 19. Prone reflex inhibiting posture with full extension.

Heel-sitting: spine extended, arms stretched forward and the head down between them. The therapist can vibrate the spine, or lower ribs (see Fig. 4).

When voicing has been facilitated in these basic reflex inhibiting postures, the therapist can try to get it in more difficult ones. She needs to be careful not to put the child into postures that he has not fully mastered in his physical therapy. For example, no attempt should be made to get him to voice in a sitting position until he is well adjusted to such a position without voicing.

Gradually, as a result of having his voice facilitated for him in a variety of different postures, the child begins to *hear* and *feel* it himself. He becomes aware of the way it changes in rhythm, pitch, length and volume under the hands of the therapist, and he delights in this new experience. As his confidence grows, the therapist is able to stimulate him less and less until finally, he is producing voice under his own control and will.

BREATHING AND VOICE

At first his voice may be weak. Hardy (37), in a study of

lung volume of children with cerebral palsy, found that their inspiratory capacities and expiratory reserves were considerably less than those of normal children. He suggests that this may be due to the weakness or paralysis of their expiratory musculature, or to the fact that in many cases, it is involuntarily opposed by the inspiratory musculature. In an attempt to correct this latter condition and to increase the volume of air, Wilson (88) used an "Electro-Lung," an apparatus which gives alternate electrical stimulation to the diaphragmatic and abdominal muscles. When tried on eight athetoid children, this apparatus was found to have been successful in superimposing a more normal respiratory pattern on the former abnormal one, and in increasing the patient's vital air capacity.

In the approach to cerebral palsy that we are describing, however, breathing is not separated from voicing. The two are practised simultaneously, and no breathing exercises as such are given. At all times the attention of the patient is drawn to voicing, that is, to breathing out, rather than to breathing in. The reason for this is, as we have already pointed out, that with cerebral palsied patients inspiration is associated with extensor spasticity. This is in accordance with the reflex behaviour of the normal infant. As he takes a deep breath he extends his whole body, and traces of this behaviour still remain with the normal adult. For example, as Marland (57) points out, we can all take a deep breath more easily if we stretch out our arms and extend our necks and spine backwards, as in yawning. When a cerebral palsied patient takes in such a deep breath he is liable to become fixed in an extensor spasm, and be unable to breath out again to make a sound. To a lesser degree, a deep breath out is apt to produce flexor spasticity in a cerebral palsied patient, and he is unable to breathe in. If a patient with predominant flexor spasticity lies on his abdomen, a position that increases his flexor spasticity, he will have great difficulty in breathing in.

ABNORMAL BREATHING AND PHONATION

At this point, a clear distinction needs to be made between the normal movements that we may use to facilitate normal voicing, and the child's former abnormal movements associated with abnormal voicing and speech.

Before receiving treatment the child's motor behaviour, including his vocalization, was dominated by his primitive reflex patterns of movement. This means that the only way he could force himself to voice was by making an abnormal movement of his body, which naturally resulted in abnormal vocalization. In other words, his breathing and vocalization were fused with his general motor behaviour, and he was unable to move one without the other. Marland (57) illustrates this point when she describes moving a severe spastics' head backward and forward. No matter how much the rhythm of these movements was varied, it was found that the breathing invariably followed this rhythm. For example, every time the neck was extended backwards there were little gasps of inspiration, followed by expiration as the head was moved forward.

The aim of the speech therapist in this approach is to dissociate the patient's speech behaviour from this abnormal motor behaviour. This, we believe, can be achieved through the use of reflex inhibiting postures, for when the patient is fully adjusted to these postures his respiratory musculature, free from spasticity, begins to work normally. As a result, he produces a greater volume of air with a consequent strengthening of vocal tone. He is no longer in danger of an extensor spasm when he breathes in, or a flexor spasm when he breathes out, because he is put into postures which favour neither total extension nor total flexion. For example, in a prone position we are careful to extend the spine fully and stretch the arms up above the head, which prevents flexor spasticity. In a "heel-sitting" position we give him a blend of extension and flexion by extending the spine and arms and flexing the hips, a posture that is the exact reverse of his habitual one. If vocalization still does not come as freely and easily as we would like, it can be facilitated by moving the child in a *normal* way while he still maintains his basic reflex inhibiting posture. It needs to be clearly understood that this normal movement and voicing is totally different from the child's former abnormal movements and abnormal voicing.

REVERSE BREATHING

If, in spite of a reflex inhibiting posture a reverse breathing pattern still persists, we believe that it can be corrected manually by the therapist. Or an apparatus, such as the "Electro-Lung" could be used, as children often enjoy this type of activity once they become accustomed to it. If it is used in this approach, however, the patient must be encouraged to phonate as he breathes out.

Research has shown that at the moment when many cerebral palsied patients are trying to talk they are, in actual fact, "inhaling" with their chests. This, of course, is the exact reverse of the normal breathing pattern. During inhalation we contract the thoracic muscles and relax the abdominal muscles, and carry out the reverse procedure during exhalation and phonation.

The first step in changing the reverse breathing pattern of the cerebral palsied patient is for the speech therapist to prevent the contraction of the thoracic muscles during exhalation and phonation, and at the same time, facilitate the contraction of the abdominal muscles. She can carry this out by using her two hands, preventing with one and facilitating with the other. She should only use her hands in this way when the patient is breathing out and voicing, and she should try to establish a rhythmic pattern of a quicker inhalation and a longer exhalation and phonation.

When the child is no longer inhaling with his thoracic muscles as he voices, the therapist can begin to facilitate the relaxation of these muscles during exhalation, together with the contraction of the abdominal muscles. As the normal respiratory pattern begins to establish itself, the therapist can use her hands less until the child is breathing normally under his own muscular control. The therapist needs to watch very carefully and at the first sign of a return to his abnormal breathing and voicing pattern she needs to use her hands to correct it once again.

VOICE QUALITY

She also needs to listen to the quality of the patient's voice. Goldschmidt (31) believes that a hoarseness in the voice is generally allied to flexor spasticity, and that it can be alleviated by the inhibition of this spasticity. For example, if a cerebral palsied child is put into a prone position and allowed to lie in his habitual posture he will have great difficulty in breathing in, and if he is able to vocalize his voice is likely to be hoarse. However, if he is put into a prone reflex inhibiting posture, the extension of his spine and arms will free him of flexor spasticity, so that his breathing and voice will become more normal.

We believe that the quality of the cerebral palsied patient's voice is very much affected by the position of his shoulders, neck, head and jaw. If he is attempting to voice when he is in his habitual posture, he will do so with associated movements of the rest of his body, and the quality of his voice, if he is able to produce it at all, will be abnormal. It is likely to be either very weak and breathy, or it will be forced and grating, probably initiated by a glottic spasm. If he is well adjusted to a reflex inhibiting posture with a consequent normal position of the shoulders, neck, head and jaw, he will be able to vocalize without effort, and the quality of his voice will be normal. If, after a short period of vocalizing in this way, he begins to show associated movements in other parts of his body, with a consequent deterioration in the quality of his voice, phonation must be stopped. Abnormal phonation, which will only lead to abnormal speech, must not be allowed. Instead, the therapist should either put the patient into an easier reflex inhibiting posture, or help him to adjust better to the one he is in.

NASALITY

A nasal voice quality is one of the problems that the speech therapist sometimes has to contend with in treating a cerebral palsied patient. This is usually due to the spasticity of the muscles of the soft palate which results in an inadequate velopharangeal closure. As a result of this, the air escapes through the patient's nose as he speaks instead of being directed through the mouth.

In one of the few studies on this subject, Dawes (18) reports that 13 per cent of 225 children with cerebral palsy had velopharyngeal closure problems affecting their speech. Hardy (37) quotes a study of forty-one children with cerebral palsy in which 39 per cent were found to have this difficulty.

Again, we believe that the nasality of the patient's vocal tone will be greatly improved by the inhibition of his reflex activity (by means of an R. I. P.) and the consequent temporary elimination of his spasticity. The therapist needs to pay special attention to the patient's shoulders, neck, head and jaw, for the position of these will be found to affect the nasality or non-nasality of his voice. For example, a posture in which the patient's head is tipped back goes far towards eliminating his nasality, for in such a posture the soft palate tends to approximate the correct position. A supine position with the therapist's arm extending the patient's dorsal spine, and his head hanging back, is an easy one with which to begin. The patient's legs can either be extended, or if he was a severe case with strong extensor spasms, they could be flexed over the end of the plinth (see Fig. 17).

The most difficult position would be with the head flexed forward for, in this position, it is easier for the air to escape through the nasal passages, probably due to the position of the tongue. If we ourselves try to vocalize, first, with our heads flexed forward, and then back, we will notice the difference in the nasality or nonnasality of our voices. Therefore, in dealing with this problem in cerebral palsied children, the therapist needs to work from the easiest towards the most difficult position, devising as many different reflex inhibiting postures as she can enroute.

EMOTIONAL STIMULATION

As the patient develops the ability to produce voice at will, in a number of different reflex inhibiting postures, the therapist needs to give special attention to training him to do so under conditions of greater emotional pressure. We believe that this is the step that a great many cerebral palsied children fail to take, with the result that they are only able to vocalize under the easiest and least pressurized of situations. If they have the potential to learn to speak and consequently communicate with others, they must be conditioned to cope with the pressures of ordinary living.

We have already described the technique of psychological desensitization in a previous chapter, and we only wish to emphasize here that it needs to be used systematically and consistently in connection with voicing. The ability to vocalize under conditions of pressure is the key to speech, and without it the child's speech will be of no great benefit to him. At this important point in the speech therapy of the cerebral palsied child we believe that the therapist needs to raise the child's tolerance level of disturbing outside influences by gradually introducing them into the therapy situation in the way we described in connection with sucking and biting.

VOWEL SOUNDS

At this stage the voicing should be confined to vowel sounds only, and it should follow roughly, but not rigidly, the normal developmental pattern. Sometimes a cerebral palsied child will produce a sound that is not in accordance with this pattern, but the therapist should follow his lead and let him make the ones that come easiest to him. Success is all she wants for him.

In Irwin's (47) study of the sounds of the new-born infant that we have already mentioned, he found that "a" sound, as in "hat" was the predominant one, and that an overwhelming majority of the crying sounds were front vowel sounds. In most cases, the cerebral palsied child also finds the front vowel sounds easier to produce than the back ones, and "a" is also often the first sound he produces. This can be followed by such sounds as "e" as in "bed," and "u" as in "but." The sound of "ee" as in "bee," and "i" as in "it" are sometimes difficult to get. This may be because in the production of an "ee" sound the back of the tongue makes a slight upward movement independently of the jaw, and the child may not yet have reached the developmental stage of being able to make such a dissociated movement. The sound of "a" as in "made" is an "extensor" sound, in that it is associated with an extensor spasm, the head being flung back and the lips drawn apart. For this reason then, it should be avoided with patients who, to begin with, have too much extensor spasticity. It is also a diphthong which makes it difficult for the child as it calls for the raising of the back of the tongue in the second half of the sound, and this may be too difficult for him at this initial stage. In general, dipthongs, such as "ow" as in "cow," and "oy" as in "boy," and triphthongs, such as "our" and "higher" are the most difficult vowel sounds for the cerebral palsied patient as they entail a changing tongue and lip position, and this coordination often remains difficult for a long time. The back vowel sounds of "o" as in "toe," "oo" as in "boot," and "aw" as in "caw" seem relatively easy to pronounce, provided that at first the child is helped to form his lips into the right positions.

PHONATION AND A LOOSE JAW

When a patient is able to vocalize at will the therapist needs to ensure that he keeps a loose jaw as he does so. We have already mentioned that the ability to move the jaw quickly and easily is one of the essentials of good articulation, and we described the way in which the therapist could train the patient to be able to do this. These movements were practised prior to vocalization. Now he needs to be trained to make the same movements *as he vocalizes*. A cerebral palsied child will find this a great deal more difficult. As soon as he begins to voice he is likely to forget to move his jaw, and it will be held rigidly in an abnormal position (usually with a deviation to the side of the greatest spasticity). If he is allowed to do this every time he vocalizes, he will never acquire the ability to move quickly and easily from one jaw position to another, as we do in normal speech. Therefore, the therapist needs to spend some time training the patient to combine the jaw movements he learned before with his new skill of voluntary phonation.

We believe that Froeschel's method of vocalized chewing is helpful for cerebral palsied patients with a severe speech involvement. In describing this method, Sittig (80) points out that it is based "on the obvious fact that chewing is one of the functions of those organs which produce speech." Therefore, she continues, since only one set of muscles and nerves serve the movements of both chewing and speaking, these functions, which can be performed at the same time, must be identical. We do not feel ourselves to be in complete agreement with these deductions, but have found that encouraging a cerebral palsied child to vocalize, as he chews, is a relatively easy way of establishing an association between phonation and jaw movements. If, at a later date, a severely handicapped child finds it easier to carry over these vocalized chewing movements into speech, we feel that he should be allowed to do so. For such a child will probably only be able to move his tongue with his jaw as in chewing, and may never be able to move it independently of his jaw as we do in normal speech. Thus "chewing his words," as advocated by Froeschels, may be the easiest form of speech for him, and for this reason, should be encouraged by the speech therapist. It must be combined with reflex inhibition, that is, the child must not be allowed to revert to his former abnormal postures and movements as he chews and speaks.

However, we do not advocate the use of this method with milder cases who, with training, can develop the ability to move the tongue independently of the jaw as is required in normal speech. If such a patient is not able to move his jaw as he vocalizes, the therapist should facilitate small, quick movements for him. Following the same procedure as before, she should gradually facilitate the movements less and less so that, without a direct request being made, the child begins to make them for himself. Having learned to do this in one body position, it needs to be practiced in as many others as possible, particularly in the *sitting position,* for it is in this position that he will ultimately do most of his talking. It also needs to be practiced under an increasing amount of emotional pressure. In short, we believe that the speech therapist should be prepared to spend a great deal of time in helping the child to acquire this skill under different physical and psychological conditions. For if he can learn to vocalize and keep a loosely moving jaw even under some pressure, he will have greatly increased his chances of being able to do the same when he begins to speak.

SUSTAINED TONE

As the child's confidence in his ability to voice increases he needs to be encouraged, first to make long and sustained sounds, and second, to change from one vowel sound to another on one exhalation. This is in preparation for the time when he will be speaking in phrases and sentences. The voice, of course, must be sustained without effort. If the patient suddenly blocks when exhaling and voicing, the therapist may be able to release him by a change in her own emotional tone. By a greater lightness or gaiety she can often reduce his tension, and so remove his block. If this does not work, a little vibration applied at the point where the blocking seems to occur, that is, where she observes a sudden fixation of movement, will almost certainly release him.

Changing from one vowel sound to another is important for the cerebral palsied patient, for this is the very essence of speech. At first he finds this hard as he is apt to fixate in one position. The therapist can help him to overcome this difficulty by first, facilitating the movements for him, and then gradually encouraging him to take over and make them for himself. As soon as he is able to make a transition from one sound to another with little help from the therapist, she can begin to introduce some rising and falling inflections into the sounds. For example:

"oo   oo"   "oh   ah"
        ee"   "ah   oo"   "oo

The aim here is to train the child to make as many vowel changes as he can on one exhalation (with varying inflections), while keeping the tone as sustained as possible.

RHYTHMIC PATTERNS OF VOICING

When the patient has acquired the ability to produce a sustained tone on one exhalation, he needs to be trained to interrupt this momentarily, and then start it again. So much of normal speech consists of stopping and starting that the sooner the cerebral palsied child learns to do this the better. Again, we have found that the therapist can facilitate this skill. By vibrating the diaphragm or larynx in rhythmic patterns of voicing and pauses, such as "ha-la-ha" and "ho-ho," she can make it possible for him to experience this sensation. At first she will have to do these more complicated movements for him, but as his confidence in his own ability grows, and he gains more control of his speech mechanism, he will be able to do more for himself. However, if a child is unable to do this, or indeed any of the movements that the speech therapist is trying to facilitate, it is unwise to let him go on trying for too long. Effort will only produce an abnormal response, and this is not what we want. In general, it is always best to abandon the attempt if the response does not come reasonably quickly and normally, and for the time being, return to any of the previous activities in which he has been successful. Later on, another attempt can be made.

LEARNING TO LISTEN

When the patient is able to vocalize at will and to make a variety of different vowel sounds, he is ready for another important phase of the treatment. He needs to be taught *to listen*.

Cerebral palsied patients, particularly those who have been frustrated by their lack of speech, are so often excited by their newly-acquired ability to vocalize that their attention is entirely focussed on "sending," and not at all on "receiving." Even if the therapist asks such a patient to listen and to copy the sounds she is making, he simply does not *receive* her. He is not wishing to be uncooperative, but his mind is busy planning the sounds he is about *to send*. Therefore, if the patient is old enough and intelligent enough to understand, it is good policy at this point in the proceedings to take the time to explain, as simply as possible, the importance of *listening*. Once a patient really grasps that the success of his sending depends on his ability to receive, a major victory has been scored.

There are two aspects of listening that are of special importance for the cerebral palsied patient. They are both closely related. First, he needs to be trained to listen to other people in order to copy the sounds they make and so improve his own speech. The speech therapist uses this aspect of listening at all times in her treatment. Secondly, he needs to be trained to listen to the sounds that he himself makes, and to evaluate and compare them with the sounds made by other people.

Van Riper and Irwin (85) make the point that in the early stages of speech learning the auditory feedback plays the dominant role in determining the correctness, or otherwise, of a word or sound. They describe the process by which a child learns to say a word in this way: "At first he must compare the self-hearing of his own utterance with the sounds that come from his parents' mouths. If they match and he is rewarded, the kinesthetic or tactual echoes or messages from his tongue position at that moment tend to become vivid and important. Soon the kinesthetic or tactual feedback is sufficiently stabilized to serve as the dominant control for speech, and the ear feedback, though still present, takes a secondary role."

We are in full agreement with this description of the process of speech learning. As the normal child uses these feedback circuits to correct his first stumbling attempts to articulate, so the cerebral palsied child must learn to use them too. With him it will be a much slower process, and at all times he will need the help and encouragement of the speech therapist, but if he has the ability to learn to speak, these self-corrective procedures must be helped to function. At the stage of therapy we have been discussing we are only concerned with the auditory feedback, for he has not yet started to use his lips and tongue to make consonant sounds. At the next stage of the treatment when the therapist begins to facilitate babbling and real words we will be stressing the importance of the kinesthetic or tactual feed-back.

Chapter VIII

ARTICULATION, LANGUAGE AND FLUENCY PROBLEMS

Accoring to Hipps (40), normal children learn basically by (1) imitation; (2) trial and error; (3) repetitive efforts, and (4) sometimes reason and insight. He goes on to stress that, in spite of their brain damage, cerebral palsied children also learn fundamentally in the same way. Therefore, when we come to teach these children, we need to keep the basic principles of learning in mind and apply them practically as far as we are able.

Writing on the same subject, Ruch (74) states that the most rapid and effective learning takes place when the individual "learns by doing." This facet of learning, however, is often denied the severely handicapped cerebral palsied child at least in the initial stages. Owing to his brain damage, he is not able to control the movements of his arms and legs, if he is learning to walk, or of his lips and tongue if he is learning to talk, so that he can learn to make these movements normally. In this approach, as we have described, the therapists facilitate the movements for him. They only do this when the child's more immature behaviour has been, first, inhibited, and the movement to be facilitated is in accordance with the next stage of normal neuro-muscular development.

Returning then to our discussion of the speech therapy of the cerebral palsied child, we believe that the next step can be taken as soon as he has achieved the following: (1) He can produce a normal voice at will, without effort, and, in the case of athetoids particularly, without associated body movements.

(2) He can do this in a variety of different body positions. (3) He can voice even when under some emotional pressure. (4) He has some measure of control over the intensity and pitch of his voice. When the child is able to carry out these requirements reasonably successfully, we believe that the speech therapist can begin to facilitate babbling.

FACILITATED BABBLING

The normal baby learns to make sounds by experimenting with his lips, tongue and soft palate, so that he feels certain movements, hears certain sounds, and learns to put them together. He enjoys this feeling of creation so much that he continues practising the sounds, and gradually rings changes and modifies them into new movements and sounds.

Due to the damage to his central nervous system, the cerebral palsied child does not have the control to move his organs of speech so precisely. If he is a spastic he may find it very difficult to move his tongue and lips at all (he may move his head and shoulders instead), and if he is able to move them he does so in a very slow and clumsy way. If he is an athetoid, on the other hand, there may be too much activity in his jaw, lips and tongue. Instead of making an exact contact with the teeth ridge his tongue tip will continually over-shoot the mark, and his efforts to control will only produce greater activity in all parts of his body. The cerebral palsied child misses the experience of learning to make sounds in the normal way.

He can learn in another way. If the speech therapist moves his lips and tongue for him, he feels the movement and hears the resulting sound, and, like the normal baby, is immediately stimulated to continue making it. At first, as before, the movements will have to be facilitated for him, but as he gains more control and confidence in himself he gradually begins to take over and make them for himself.

SOUND OR SYLLABLE

The question of whether the therapist should first facilitate a sound or syllable depends on the individual child. If he has not yet begun to speak, we believe that she should facilitate a syllable rather than an isolated sound, for this is in accordance with normal speech development. When at about three months of age a normal baby begins to babble, the sounds he produces are syllables. As Greene (34) observes, "He starts with a simple 'da,' 'ya,' 'ga' or 'ba' interspersed with coos, but gradually, long repetitive strings develop." Therefore, in facilitating babbling with a cerebral palsied child who can voice, but has not yet begun to speak, the speech therapist should facilitate such syllables as these.

In treating a cerebral palsied child who has already begun to speak, however, she is faced with a different problem. Such a child may have established the habit of using a wrong sound, for instance, a "d" sound instead of a "g" sound. If this is the case, we believe it is necessary for the speech therapist to facilitate the sound and help the child to become aware of it in isolation. Van Riper (83) has stated that the mastering of a new sound so that it can be used habitually in speech has to take place at four successive levels: " (1) the isolated sound level; (2) the sound in a syllable; (3) the sound in a word, and (4) the sound in a meaningful sentence." Therefore, if the problem is that the cerebral palsied child is habitually using a wrong sound in his speech, we agree that the speech therapist should first facilitate the correct sound in isolation. Only when the child is able to produce it in isolation, and is aware of the difference between it and the incorrect sound, should the therapist combine it with a vowel sound.

The question of which consonant sound to facilitate first is a matter for experimentation with the individual child. Normal babies show slight variations in their first babbling noises, some producing the back sounds of "g" and "k" first, and some the lip sounds of "b," "m" or "w." It is wisest to start with whichever is easiest for the individual child, for above everything, his need is to succeed. Usually the voiced consonant sounds are easier for a child than their voiceless equivalents.

FACILITATING A "G" SOUND

The reflex inhibiting posture which the therapist chooses for the child depends on the particular consonant which she is trying to facilitate. For instance, if she decides to try to get the "g" sound first, it is best to have him in a supine position with the legs either flexed up on to his chest, or hanging over the end of the plinth (depending on the stage he has reached in his physical therapy). The therapist can then put one arm under the child's dorsal spine, extending it, and encourage the child to let his head fall back (see Fig. 17).

If she then encourages him to voice as she gives a series of gentle pressures well back under his chin, she will be instrumental in pushing up the back of his tongue against the palate as is required for the production of a "g" sound. At the same time she needs to make the sound herself, and with this double-barrelled stimulation, he is likely to produce it without too much difficulty. The "g" sound is sometimes one of the easiest sounds to facilitate with a cerebral palsied patient, perhaps because he often seems to be more aware of his throat and the back of his tongue than he is of the front of his palate and his tongue tip. Also, from the point of view of his neuro-muscular development the cerebral palsied child may well find "g" a relatively easy sound to produce because it calls for a more gross movement of the back of the tongue than, for instance, the sound of "l" which calls for a finer movement of the tongue tip involving more precise coordination.

If the therapist is unable to get a satisfactory "g" sound in the way just described, another method is suggested. If a little water is poured into the mouth of any normal person lying in a supine position, the back of the tongue immediately rises against the velum in a reflex movement to prevent choking. This method can be used, with the utmost caution, with the cerebral palsied child for, starting at first with just a few drops, the water will stimulate the raising of the back of the tongue, and so make it easier for the therapist to facilitate the "g" and "k" sounds.

As soon as the therapist has achieved a satisfactory "g" sound, she should try for it again, but this time in a more modified reflex inhibiting posture. For instance, she could remove her arm from under the child's dorsal spine, so that his head is no longer tipped back, but is in a normal mid-line position, and then try to facilitate the sound. Once the child has the idea of the sound that is required of him, and has heard himself make it successfully, it can usually be facilitated in many different positions without too much difficulty. Gradually the therapist reduces the stimulation, and encourages the child to take over the movement for himself, and if she makes the transition from *her* control to *his* control smoothly, he is likely to take over surprisingly quickly.

When the cerebral palsied child who has not yet begun to speak can babble "ga-ga-ga" with very little help from the therapist, she can begin to introduce a variation of vowel sounds. It is likely that the sound of "a" as in "hat" (being one of the early sounds) will be an easy one for him, but she should bring in as many different ones as possible and practice changing from one to another. At first she may have to facilitate the babbling for him again, using her hands to help him with either the consonant or vowel sound, or even both, if necessary. A child always enjoys this experience, for it amuses him to hear and feel himself making sounds over which, at first, he has no control. As soon as the facilitated babbling begins to come easily and smoothly in the easiest reflex inhibiting posture, the therapist should go through the usual process of gradually allowing the child to take over control until he is able to babble in this position with little, if any, help from her. This same procedure needs to be repeated in a variety of different body positions, one of these, of course, being the sitting position. It may be more difficult for him to control his head in this position than it is in prone or supine lying, yet this position, as has already been pointed out, is the one in which he will do most of his talking. At this stage also every effort should be made to raise his tolerance level to emotional pressure. He needs to be systematically trained to continue his babbling under emotional stimulation, so that, when the time comes for him to produce his first words, and later on, to combine them into short sentences, he will be conditioned to speak under the pressures of every day living.

FACILITATING LIP SOUNDS

If the therapist decides to start with the lip sounds of "b," "p" or "w," a supine reflex inhibiting posture is usually the easiest, but this time the head should be allowed to lie in the normal midline position. By this time, some children are so well-conditioned that when the therapist uses her fingers to bring the upper and lower lips together in a series of quick, light movements, and produces voice herself, they will begin to voice with her, and the resultant sound will be a "b." As many cerebral palsied children have a tendency to be nasal, it is wiser to facilitate the lip sounds of "b," "p" or "w" rather than the nasal sound of "m." Once they become aware of their lips and that they can be brought together to make a sound, they are likely to produce the sound of "m" on their own without any additional practice. While she is facilitating the "b," "p" and "w" sounds, the therapist should do all in her power to make the child as aware of his lips as possible by gently manipulating them, both with and without voicing, and by rubbing them lightly with her finger.

FACILITATING TONGUE-TIP SOUNDS

Before attempting to facilitate any tongue-tip sounds such as "t," "d" or "l," the therapist again needs to make the child aware of his tongue tip. She can do this by touching it gently with her finger or tongue depressor, by having him lick a candy or ice cream cone held for him, or by sticking a soft candy on to his teeth ridge and, holding his teeth a little apart, have him try to lick it with his tongue tip.

As soon as the child has some awareness of the tip of his tongue, the therapist needs to attempt to facilitate "d" and "t" sounds. For this she must help the child adjust to a position in which his head is flexed forward, for in this position, the tongue tip is more likely to approximate the correct position, that is, raised towards the teeth ridge. If the therapist pushes up under the child's chin as he voices, and makes a "d" sound herself, she may be successful in getting it from him. The following reflex inhibiting postures could be used in facilitating a "d" or "t" sound:

Sitting: with legs hanging over the end of the plinth, arms supporting the trunk, and with the head flexed forward (see Fig. 18).

Supine: (if the above position is too difficult) with legs flexed over the end of the plinth, and with the head flexed forward by the therapist (see Fig. 14).

Prone: with the trunk supported on flexed elbows and the head flexed forward or held straight (see Fig. 15).

The facilitation of such sounds as "f," "v," "th" and "l" are relatively easy, for it is necessary to assume well-defined mouth positions in order to say them. This makes it easier for both the therapist and the child. She can show him what mouth position is required, and then facilitate it for him so that he feels it for himself. Usually these sounds do not represent any great difficulty.

MOTOR KINESTHETIC METHOD

It will be apparent that the way in which sounds are facilitated in this approach to cerebral palsy bears a great similarity to the "Motor Kinesthetic" method of speech training worked out by Mrs. Edna Hill-Young. We believe that such a similarity does indeed exist. For example, in describing the Moto-Kinesthetic method, Hahn (36) notes that "it endeavours to guide the muscles of the speech apparatus into accurate movements for the production of correct sound sequences"—a description that could equally well be applied to the sound facilitation of this approach.

Again, Stinchfield Hawk (38), writing on the Moto-Kinesthetic method remarks: "The Hill-Young method of moto-sensory speech training differs from other methods in use, in that it does not depend upon auditory or visual stimuli alone to initiate speech movements. The teacher actually sets the pattern for the child, giving suggestions to the muscle groups by muscular and kinesthetic sensation, so that the child knows definitely by pressure exerted at the base of the tongue on the outside of the throat, that the tongue moves backward and upward for "k" and "g," and "ng" sounds, for example. While at first it may be necessary to use the tongue depressor to stimulate the tongue to rise for the "t," "d" and "n" sounds contacting the alveolar process just in back of the upper front teeth: after a time (varying according to the sound desired), a light pressure above the upper lip in mid-line, on the outside, is all that is necessary to give the child the suggestion that will enable him to execute the proper tongue-end movement."

It will be seen that the facilitating of sounds we have described and the Moto-Kinesthetic method have much in common. They both attempt to reinforce the auditory and visual stimulation by giving the child the feeling of the movement, believing that the kinesthetic feed-back is a potent factor in establishing speech habits. Van Riper and Irwin (85), it will be remembered, also stress that the kinesthetic feedback of a sound or word quickly becomes the dominant control in speech.

In accordance with the concept of reflex inhibition, more is done in positioning the cerebral palsied patient before sounds are facilitated than is done in the Moto-Kinesthetic method. Greater attention is also probably paid to the patient's general body condition, rather than only to the movements of his speech mechanism. The sound facilitation we have been describing was evolved specifically for cerebral palsied patient in this particular approach, whereas the Moto-Kinesthetic method, we believe, was primarily evolved for normal children with defective speech. However, it has been used with cerebral palsied patients. In writing on the subject of cerebral palsy, Hill-Young and Stinchfield Hawk (91) state that the Moto-Kinesthetic method has been found to be more successful with these patients than therapy which made use of visual and auditory stimulation.

SPONTANEOUS BABBLING

As soon as most of the easier consonant sounds have been facilitated in this way, and the child has had some experience, first, of facilitated babbling, and then of being able to babble under his own control in the therapy situation, he is likely to begin babbling spontaneously on his own at other times. At this stage of the therapy, parents often report that when the child is in bed, either first thing in the morning, or at night, they hear him beginning to make the babbling sounds of a young baby. Here the cerebral palsy child is simply following the normal developmental pattern and practicing his newly-acquired sounds on his own even as the young baby does. Parents should be warned not to go in and interrupt this most important practice period, for it is a necessary stage in speech development that precedes the appearance of true words. The ability to babble freely and easily depends on the degree to which the child's speech is involved in his general condition, and also on his emotional problems (if any), and his adjustment to them.

Any sign of abnormality in the babbling, such as a forced voice, grimacing, or babbling accompanied by a return to the child's former abnormal movement patterns should be stopped. Normal movements, such as the therapist may have used in facilitating voicing, can be combined with babbling, for this is in accordance with normal speech development. The normal baby moves his arms and legs as he babbles, and later on, this ability to move as he vocalizes will enable him to speak as he performs functional movements such as walking, and dressing himself. Only the cerebral palsied child with minimal brain damage is likely to reach this stage. If he does, he will need the combined help of the physical therapist, the occupational therapist, and the speech therapist to acquire these skills.

INTRODUCING VARIATIONS

So far, the babbling will have consisted of the consonant sound placed initially before the vowel sound, as in "ba-ba-ba" and "ga-ga-ga." When the child's babbling in this pattern has become fairly well established, the therapist could introduce a variation by putting the consonant sound medially, starting with whichever one the child finds the easiest. For example, she can facilitate the sounds of "aga- aga- aga," or "aba- aba- aba." When the child has mastered this, she can try putting the consonant sound finally as in "ag - ag - ag" or "ab - ab - ab," so that the child has the experience of using it in all positions in preparation for the pronunciation of real words. As soon as the child has had a little success in this, words which have the same arrangement of vowel and consonant sounds may be introduced into the babbling. At first, it is probably best not to associate too much meaning to these babbled words until the child has mastered the technique of saying them. If in the initial stages they are used too meaningfully the child will become excited and so be unable to execute the relatively fine movements required in their production. This follows the normal developmental speech pattern for a normal baby will babble "da-da-da" or "mumumum" before he relates these words to specific persons. When the cerebral palsied child has mastered the technique of saying certain words, then he can be encouraged to use them meaningfully.

FACILITATING THE SIBILANTS

The acquisition of the remaining consonant sounds, such as the sibilants and "r" sounds, are more difficult for the therapist to facilitate, as they call for a less easily-defined mouth position, and for more subtle coordinations. By this time the child will have much greater confidence in his ability, however, and, as a result of the facilitation of the easier consonant sounds, he will have acquired the ability to make more selective movements of his speech mechanism. Sometimes the use of straws is very helpful for the facilitation of sibilant sounds such as "s," "sh" and "ch." If the straw is placed in front of the child's closed teeth, and he is encouraged to hiss down it, while the therapist stimulates him by making the required sound herself, he very often produces the "s" sound surprisingly quickly and easily. The advantage of a straw is that the child himself hears his own breath escaping through it, and this highlights the fact that for this sound the breath must come down the center of the tongue and out between his two front teeth. A cerebral palsied child seems to find it easier to let his breath out at each side of his tongue rather than down the middle, with the result that when he attempts to make any sibilant sound he does so with a strong lateral lisp. This can be illustrated for him very clearly by encouraging him to let his breath out as he habitually does, that is laterally, and holding two straws one on each side of his mouth to catch the escaping breath; and then by contrast, holding one straw in front of his closed teeth and encouraging him to hiss down the center of his tongue and out through the straw. Some children may find it easier to achieve the "s" sound first, and others the "sh" sound, but as soon as one sibilant sound is achieved it usually does not take him long to acquire the others.

LANGUAGE DEVELOPMENT

We need to remember, however, that the normal child produces his first words, begins to put them together, and use them for communication before he is able to say all his consonant sounds correctly. Indeed, as we know, some children do not master these completely until they are from six to seven years of age or even older. Therefore, as soon as the cerebral palsied child has gained some control over his speech mechanism through the practice of, first, facilitated, and then spontaneous babbling, and has perhaps produced his first few words, we believe that the therapist should turn her attention to the development of language.

It is natural that language, that is the ability to communicate and understand others through the use of spoken words, develops more slowly in cerebral palsied than in normal children, but it follows the same developmental pattern. We have already quoted research showing that cerebral palsied children produce single words at approximately twenty-seven months of age, whereas normal children produce them at approximately twelve months of age. From the same source, Denhoff and Holden (19), we find that cerebral palsied children produce two-word sentences at about thirty-seven months, while normal children produce them at about twenty-four months. Byrne (12) studying the same subject, found that the median age at which a group of seventy-four cerebral palsied children produced three-word sentences was seventy-eight months, while normal children produced them at about thirty months. This represents a delay of approximately one year in the production of single words and two-word sentences, and a delay of four years in the production of three-word sentences. In breaking down these figures still further, Byrne reports an interesting difference between the speech development of the spastic and athetoid group. It was found that the spastics developed words and sentences earlier than the athetoids. For example, the spastics in the group produced two-word sentences at thirty months and three-word sentences at sixty months. The athetoids, on the other hand, produced two-word sentences at fifty-four months, and the "median for three-word sentences could not be computed because more than one half were not yet using them."

When we come to the question of helping the cerebral palsied child to learn to communicate we are confronted with a variety of different theories of language development. From these we have selected the ones which, in our opinion, are the most fundamental, and if applied, will help the child most effectively.

THE NEUROPHYSIOLOGICAL APPROACH

Penfield and Roberts (68) believe that the development of oral language is dependent on the formation in the central nervous system of three types of neuronal patterns which represent what they call the "conceptual," "sound," and "verbal" units. For example, the child would acquire the word "milk" in the following way: by repeatedly experiencing "milk" he eventually establishes a neuronal pattern which represents the idea of milk. At the same time, by repeatedly hearing the word "milk" he also eventually establishes a neuronal pattern which represents the sound of the word "milk." By virtue of the frequent association between the idea of milk and the sound of the word, a reciprocal reflex connection is made between the two, with the result that a verbal unit becomes established which represents the spoken word "milk."

Penfield's research indicates that the first step in the development of oral language consists of perceptual experiences, and that without the growth of neuronal patterns (representing these experiences), it is impossible for a child to produce a word meaningfully. This we believe has special implications for the cerebral palsied child who, as a result of his physical disabilities, has been prevented from acquiring many of the perceptual experiences of the normal child. Therefore, as soon as the cerebral palsied child has reached the stage of language development, we suggest that the speech therapist should plan a program of perceptual training with the object of heightening and exciting the child's powers of perception. Here the therapist needs to work first in the area that is of particular interest to the individual child. Usually this is himself, for few cerebral palsied children have had the opportunity to develop fields of interests outside of themselves. By putting into effect the principles of word-learning, as formulated by Penfield, the therapist should endeavour to increase the child's awareness of the different parts of his body with their associated names. Starting from this central point the perceptual training should extend outwards to include the child's family, food, clothing, home, and so out into his environment. In addition to this objective perceptual training, Mysak (63) suggests that materials should be used that excite the child's visual, auditory, tactual, kinesthetic, gustatory and olfactory sensations: and that he should be asked to imagine an object's colour, texture, taste and smell. We are in full agreement with these suggestions, and feel that they could play an important part in helping the cerebral palsied child to develop his language ability.

THE IMITATION THEORY

Obviously, imitation through listening is an important part of the language learning process. If it were not, deaf children would learn to speak as readily as children with normal hearing, which demonstrably is not the case. According to Van Riper (83), the most effective way for an adult to get a child to imitate her, is by first imitating the child. This, of course, is contrary to generally accepted beliefs, but when we come to examine the situation we must admit it seems to make sense!

Van Riper believes that a baby's imitation is based on the desire to perpetuate a stimuli that interested and intrigued him. If he did not repeat it, his memory span being very short, he would immediately forget it. Thus, he repeats "da-da-da-da-da" because if he didn't, he would forget the sound. Taking advantage of this predisposition to repeat an interesting stimulus, the adult should join in with the child as soon as he starts his repetitive string of babbled sounds. This usually has the effect of stopping the child, while he observes the adult. After a pause, however, he resumes his babbling and is again imitated by the adult, and the same procedure is repeated. It is not long before the pause between the adult's imitation of the child and the child's resumption of his activity becomes so abbreviated that the child begins to act in response to the adult's stimulation. Van

Riper (83) states that this training should be continued until the child "responds consistently with eager repetition whenever the parent has interrupted vocal play by imitating his vocalizations." It can be readily seen that once this pattern of imitation has been established between an adult and child, the adult is in a very favourable position for helping the child to acquire real words and sentences.

However, the importance of imitation in the development of language it not considered to be quite as great as it used to be. Shelton, Arndt and Miller (78) appear to sum up the present feeling in the following words: "The relationship of imitation to various principles of learning apparently has not been determined, nor have the circumstances been determined under which imitation occurs. Before language acquisition is attributed primarily to imitation, the subject should receive intense investigation."

THE AUTISM THEORY

Mowrer (61), believing that the relationship of imitation to speech learning calls for further investigation, has propounded a new theory that has a bearing on this subject. This is the so-called "autism" theory of language learning. It is based on the belief that emotional states have an important relationship to an individual's capacity to remember and learn. Therefore, in relating this belief to the first stages of word-learning, we could say that if the word said, for example, by the mother, produces a positive emotional reaction in the child, he will be stimulated to make the same sound and to retain it. If, on the other hand, the word said by the mother produces an unfavourable or negative reaction in the child he will not make any attempt to reproduce it or retain it.

Mowrer developed this theory from working with talking birds. He found that the basis for teaching them words was to make *pets* of them, so that they always anticipated his appearance with eagerness and pleasure. If he then always said a word, such as "hello," as he appeared, the word became for the bird a *good* sound with pleasant associations attached to it. According to Mowrer (61), the next step followed quickly for the bird being "vocally versatile" made random attempts to produce the sound, one of which happened to approximate it. This brought an instant feedback of pleasant memories with the result that the bird made the effort to repeat and perfect it. The more closely the bird matched the sound, the greater satisfaction it experienced.

This in essence is the "autism" theory of language learning —"autism," according to Van Riper (83) referring to the "self-rewarding aspect of the process." We believe that it can be applied effectively in the first stages of word learning with both normal and cerebral palsied children. In other words, if the therapist establishes a warm and friendly relationship with the child so that he anticipates his session with her with eager pleasure, the first step in word-learning will have taken place. If she then associates a word or short sentence with this pleasant feeling, the child will be stimulated to reproduce this sound and practice it in order to experience the pleasant feedback of memories and associations.

These then are a few of the theories of language development which, we believe, practically applied are effective in helping the cerebral palsied child to talk. Before discussing other ways in which he can be helped to become more fluent, we will describe, briefly, the different phases of language development.

THE SEQUENTIAL PROCESS OF LANGUAGE DEVELOPMENT

There appear to be three phases of language development, each having its own particular characteristic, and yet each merging into and blending with the other.

The characteristic of the first phase is percept formation, that is, the recognition of objects and activities, and the learning of words with which to label them. This phase starts when the child is approximately one year of age and reaches its peak between his first and second birthdays. The characteristic of the second phase, which starts as soon as the child begins to put his words together into short sentences, is what Piaget (71) has called "egocentric" speech. The characteristic of the third phase, which starts a little later, possibly around the child's third birthday, is "socialized" speech.

According to Piaget, egocentric speech consists of vocalization in which the child repeats words or syllables, for the pleasure of talking: monologues, in which he talks to himself as though he were thinking aloud: collective monologues, in which another child is present but his point of view is never taken into account: questions and answers. Socialized speech, on the other hand, is when the child really exchanges his thoughts with others: when he criticizes others, or commands, requests, or threatens them.

From his own research Piaget estimated that 38 per cent of the child's conversation was egocentric and 62 per cent was socialized. However, subsequent research on this subject has produced a wide divergency of opinion ranging from agreement to complete disagreement (for example, McCarthy (58) reported that according to her findings only 3.6 per cent of a child's vocalizations were egocentric in nature).

The cerebral palsied child's language development will, of course, follow the same sequential pattern as the normal child, but at a much slower pace. He may not reach the period of percept formation until he is approximately twenty-seven months old, and he may not reach the stages of egocentric and socialized talking until he is from three to four years of age, or even much older. If he has the mental ability to speak, and the physical ability to control his speech mechanism, he will in due course reach both these stages. The skill of the speech therapist lies in recognizing the child's level of language development, and helping him to advance to a higher level of speech and communication.

ESTABLISHING PATTERNS OF FLUENCY

Before discussing how the therapist can help the cerebral palsied child to speak more fluently, it would be as well if we reviewed briefly the way in which the normal child becomes fluent.

Speech fluency is the inevitable result of the truly astonishing vocabulary increase that takes place between the child's second and fourth birthdays. As Greene (34) notes, at two years "a forward child may use a hundred words, at two and a half four hundred words, and at three years, eight hundred words." And he goes on acquiring, on the average, about fifty new words a month until he has passed his fourth birthday, after which the vocabulary explosion gradually eases off.

This sudden growth in the child's vocabulary coincides with his awakening interest in the world around him. He *needs* words to label the many and interesting objects he is continually finding, and to describe his new and exciting experiences. Inevitably his words begin to fall into patterns, and to make short sentences. This is particularly the case with the child who is blessed with understanding parents who provide him with a model by talking to him in short two- and three-word sentences that he can copy. It is harder for the child whose parents speak to him quickly in a nonstop adult fashion, using long and involved sentences. Such a child, unable to disentangle the speech-noise into individual words may well lapse back into jargon (for this is how it sounds to him), with the result that he will be late in acquiring the normal patterns of fluent speech. Speaking generally, it could be said that the average child begins to combine words just before his second birthday. Very shortly after this he begins to use compound sentences, and by the time he has reached his third birthday he is using complex sentences and speaking relatively fluently.

FLUENCY AND THE CEREBRAL PALSIED

The cerebral palsied child, being unable to explore his world as freely as a normal child, is not so likely to have the same rapid growth of percept formation. Owing to his physical condition he will not have the opportunity of discovering a wide range of new objects and activities requiring words to identify them. Yet, as we have seen, it is the sudden rush of new words and experiences that all but forces the normal child to begin to put his words together into first, two, and then three-word sentences. Single words are no longer adequate to express the new ideas that keep sweeping over him. The problem, then, that confronts the therapist and parents is how to help the cerebral palsied child to gain this experience, for without it he will not talk.

We believe that as soon as a cerebral palsied child has gained some control over his speech mechanism, the speech therapist and the parents (under her instruction) should embark on a systematic program of percept training, that is, in the recognition and labelling of objects and activities. This should be carried out along the lines suggested by Penfield, Van Riper and Mowrer, and continued until the child has approximately a hundred words in his vocabulary which he can recognize, reproduce and use meaningfully. (A normal child has approximately this number of words at his disposal when he begins to put them together into short sentences.)

When the cerebral palsied child has reached this level of language development he should be helped to put one or two words together. In the initial stages of word-combination the normal child uses such phrases as "all gone"; "go away"; "Kitty bye-bye," and if the cerebral palsied child is young enough he should be stimulated to use such and similar phrases. If he is older he can be taught to use the conjunction "and" to join words together. For example, "arm *and* leg," "eyes *and* nose," "bread *and* butter," and so on. All children enjoy the game of putting words together in this way. The principles of language learning we have already discussed can be used equally well in the teaching of two- and three-word sentences as in the teaching of single words.

The parents (and, of course, the therapist) can help a great deal at this stage. If they make a point of always speaking to the child slowly and clearly, in short two- and three-word sentences, they are giving him a pattern on which to model his own speech. We believe that if the cerebral palsied child (with a speech potential) is spoken to in this way it is possible to save him from the jargon phase of speech development that a great many normal children go through between eighteen and thirty months of age. It is our belief that this phase is often simply the result of a child having his ears bombarded by a barrage of nonstop, indistinct adult speech. To the child it simply sounds like jargon, and so, wishing to speak like the adults, he too uses jargon. The interesting point is that some children do not go through this stage. Their speech progresses in a relatively orderly fashion from single words to two- and three-word sentences, to compound ones, and so on gradually to adult patterns of fluency with little or no hitch. This, we feel, is due to the fact that their parents did not overwhelm them with a flood of words, but always spoke to them in a way they could understand and copy. If, by parental care, jargon can be avoided for the normal child, we believe that every effort should be made to enable the cerebral palsied child to avoid it too. His speech and language development are going to be slow enough without unnecessary and added complications. If those in his immediate environment always speak to him slowly and clearly, using short words and phrases, he too, will progress from single words to sentences without being bogged down in a welter of jargon.

Every small child enjoys the rhythm and lilt of nursery rhymes and jingles, and these can be used to help the cerebral palsied child to become aware of the latent rhythm of the language he is in the process of learning. Perhaps one of the best ways of helping him to acquire the phrasing and inflections of adult speech is through the use of what has been called "parallel talking."

In describing this technique, Van Riper (83) states "the therapist must verbalize for the patient his thoughts at the moment they occur." For example, as the child is drinking milk from a cup the therapist says: "drink milk"; as he drains the last drop she says: "all gone"; and as he bangs his empty cup on the table she says, "bang, bang, bang." In other words, we try to verbalize the thoughts that enter the child's mind as his actions evoke them. The purpose is to put correctly spoken thoughts into the child's thinking, for he will not be able to speak clearly and well until he is thinking in this way. The therapists' words, matching his actions, gives him a model for speech, and the correct phrases become part, first, of his thinking, and then of his speech. This technique has been particularly successful with children and adults who, for one reason or another, are having any type of language difficulty. For this reason we believe that if it is used to describe the things the cerebral palsied child sees, hears, feels, thinks and does, it is a most effective way of helping him to establish the normal patterns of fluent speech.

This brings us to the conclusion of suggested techniques for helping the cerebral palsied child to talk. We fully realize that those children who are seriously handicapped and have a severe speech involvement are not likely to reach the final stages of therapy we have just been describing. With such children who are not destined to reach the level of neuro-muscular development necessary for the production of words and sentences, and who also may not have the intelligence to reach even the stage of percept formation, there is little the therapist can do. At the same time, that little should be done.

We have attempted to lay down a blue-print of speech therapy for the cerebral palsied child, and it is our sincere hope that every child should be helped to implement it up to the level of his individual physical and mental capacities.

Chapter IX

PSYCHOLOGICAL ASPECTS OF THE PROBLEM

WE have attempted to describe the Bobath approach to the treatment of cerebral palsy with particular reference to the part played by the speech therapist. No such discussion would be complete without mention being made of the psychological aspects of the problem. In the final analysis, these outweigh all others. Therapy, whether it be physical, occupational or speech, cannot be imposed from the outside with little consideration or understanding of the individual who is receiving it. Such therapy can only fail, or achieve very superficial success. True therapy takes place when the therapist is so attuned to the patient that she has insight into his immediate needs, and is able to devise a way of fulfilling them successfully. This can be achieved best, we believe, in the type of holistic approach we have been describing.

Here the patient is viewed as a whole. The level of his neuro-muscular development is assessed, and he is given the treatment that will inhibit his present motor behaviour and facilitate the next step for him. In the first stages when gross movements of his body have to be inhibited, and less gross ones facilitated, it is the physical therapist who will be predominant on the team. As the patient gains greater control of his movements the occupational therapist will begin to come into the picture, and teach him to do simple activities for himself. When he has some measure of control over his arms, legs and hands, the speech therapist begins to facilitate the finer movements required for speech. The treatment, following the pattern of normal development, is a systematic progression from gross to fine physical movements, with the appropriate therapist taking over at the appropriate moment. In addition to this dovetailing of treatment each therapist views the patient as a whole as she works with him on his own. In other words, she does not work exclusively with his arms and legs, or hands or jaw, but continually watches his whole body and general muscle tone. For, as she knows, as long as this is normal, his movements will be normal; but once his general condition deteriorates, he will be unable to move any part of his body in a normal way.

This, as we have seen, is the basis of the treatment we have been describing; and this cooperation between therapists must not be limited to the patient's physical difficulties. If the full potential of the treatment is to be implemented the same cooperation and understanding must also be extended to include the psychological aspects of the problem. We are treating a child, not muscles and reflex movements, and therefore, we must get to know and understand that child. To gain insight into his attitudes (towards himself, his handicap, and towards other people), we must get to know his parents and his home, for this is where his attitudes are bred.

PSYCHOLOGICAL FACTORS AND SPEECH DEVELOPMENT

Getting to know and understand the child has a special importance for the speech therapist for psychological factors are known to have a bearing on speech development. We have already quoted Hood, Shank, and Williamson (43) and Carlson (13) to show that there is often a discrepancy between the severity of a cerebral palsied child's disabilities and his actual functioning, particularly in the field of speech. Many other writers, including Pintner (72), Rutherford (75) and Palmer (66) have agreed that a child's speech performance is determined not only by the extent and severity of the brain damage, but also by psychological factors in his environment. The implication of the research is that such factors can either impede or accelerate the child's speech development.

Psychological factors in the child himself could also have an effect on his speech behaviour. Schlanger (77) in a study of the speech and language development of brain damaged children found that the longer communication habilitation is delayed, the greater the child's anxiety about such therapy, and consequently, the slower his progress. He also found that if communication was still severely limited by the time a child had reached the chronological age of seven years, such a child rarely attained a normal level of speech and language development. Although these findings are related specifically to retarded brain-damaged children, we believe that they are applicable, in a lesser degree, to cerebral palsied children with normal intelligence.

THE MOTHER AND THE CEREBRAL PALSIED CHILD

In the main, however, we believe that the psychological factors that could impede or accelerate a child's speech development are to be found in the home, and particularly in the relationship that exists between the child and its mother. A cerebral palsied child is dependent on its mother for so much longer than the normal child. In many cases he has to be bathed, dressed, fed and carried for years after the normal child is looking after himself and leading an independent life of his own. Under such circumstances, it is not surprising that the cerebral palsied child is deeply influenced by its mother's attitudes and feelings, and that they often become as much a part of him as they are of her.

When we come to study the different relationships that exist between mothers and their cerebral palsied children, we find that, in general, they seem to be based on three main attitudes. First, and probably the most common, is an attitude of overprotection. The mother completely renounces any independent life of her own and devotes herself almost exclusively to the care and welfare of the child. This reaction is understandable, for a cerebral palsied child, while affecting the life of every member of the family, drastically changes the mother's. It is only too easy for her to become utterly absorbed in him. If the child is allowed to dominate the home a state of imbalance is created that is harmful for everyone concerned, particularly the child himself. If life at home revolves around him, naturally enough, he expects the same conditions outside his home. This makes life unnecessarily hard for him, and also makes it difficult for the therapists and teachers to help him.

The second type of attitude shown by mother is probably based on feelings of resentment, or guilt, at having this problem to cope with (the over-indulgence of the child may, of course, also stem from the same feelings). In this case the mother's attitude towards the child is variable. At times she indulges him and at others her own frustration and anxiety show in her handling of him. This produces tension between them, and causes the child to show the same symptoms of anxiety and frustration which, as we have already seen, tend to increase his difficulties.

The third type of attitude is a much more objective one in that the mother, while looking after and fulfilling the child's physical and emotional needs, does not allow herself to become totally involved in his problem. She knows that he has to be physically dependent on her because of his disability, but she handles the situation in such a way that he does not also become too psychologically dependent on her. She seems to achieve this by her own mature attitude, and an instinctive realization that, in spite of his handicap, the child must follow the normal developmental pattern and reach at least some degree of independence from her. To this end she tries to have some small area of her life apart from the child and, as he grows older, tries to make it possible for him to have the same.

The child who has such a mother is lucky indeed, for she helps him develop a sense of perspective about his disorder. As he grows up he is able to view it objectively as a subject to be studied with interest, but also as one that need not engulf his whole horizon. He has physical disabilities, but apart from these he becomes aware of himself as a person with immense potentialities for growth, learning and friendship. This detached acceptance of himself destroys any vestige of self-pity, shame, resentment of any of the feelings that increase rather than lighten the individual's load. It is an attitude that, we believe, enables a handicapped person (or anyone else, for that matter) to live gracefully and happily with himself. It also helps him to live more happily with other people, for when an individual has resolved his own difficulties he begins to take a livelier interest in other people. Obviously, the ability to make friends and enjoy the company of other people will do much to enrich a cerebral palsied patient's life.

These, then, are some of the more common attitudes and relationships that develop between mothers and their cerebral palsied children. If the therapists feel that a particular relationship between a child and his mother is unsatisfactory in that it is impeding his progress, we believe that they should take steps to try to remedy this. We have found that group discussions between mothers under the direction of the pediatrician, psychologist or a therapist (whichever one is best fitted for the task) is a constructive way of dealing with this situation. It is a relief for mothers to be able to discuss their difficulties with others in a similar position, and a free exchange of ideas, under expert guidance, leads to a gradual change of attitude which is of benefit both to mother and child.

THE ROLE OF THE MOTHER

We feel that it is of the utmost importance that the mother should be brought into the therapy program. The speech therapist, in particular, needs her help. As we have already mentioned, it is the mother who first communicates (in a nonverbal way) with her baby and thereby lays the foundation for his later ability to communicate through the use of words. In her "Open Letter to the Parents of the Cerebral Palsied Child," Huber (45) stresses the importance of this early communication and the need, as the child grows older, for continuing this pleasant experience. Unless the cerebral palsied child has always enjoyed communication (even without speech) , he may not want to make the effort to learn to speak. Therefore, from the point of view of the speech therapist, the mother is a key person in her program, and should be included from the first.

A mother is often able to play a decisive role in the therapy itself. For example, it sometimes happens that a young child will be vocalizing at home, but will refuse (or be unable to do so) in the therapy room. In such a case, it is the mother who can resolve such a situation rather than the therapist. If she is left alone with the child and holds and plays with him as she does at home, he will soon begin vocalizing as he does there. This should be carried on for several sessions, so that the child becomes accustomed to vocal play in these new surroundings. Once this pattern has been established, the speech therapist can also be there, but unobstrusively, letting the mother play the leading role. When the child is accustomed to her presence he will carry on as before playing and vocalizing with his mother. Gradually, the therapist can take part in the play until the child is vocalizing as freely with her as he is with his mother. We believe that it pays to take plenty of time to resolve such a situation, particularly if it is connected with first vocalizations, for this is the basis of speech. If the therapist tries to handle the situation on her own she may create a psychological blocking that could seriously delay the child's acquisition of speech. By including the mother in the way we have described, the situation resolves itself in the easiest and most natural way.

Again, the mother can give invaluable assistance in the field of perceptual training. Huber (45), writing to parents, advises them to teach the child "to notice more things every day by means of the senses of sight, hearing, touch, smell and taste. If he must remain seated a great part of the time, place him where there is something worth looking at." The normal child can move around and by means of his five senses explore the world for himself, but the cerebral palsied child needs to have the world brought to him. No one is in a better position to do that than the mother who spends so much of her time with him, and, by doing so, she is playing a vital role in his language habilitation.

There are, of course, many times when the speech therapist will feel she will do better with the child on her own, for some children will not respond so well when their mothers are there. None the less, we feel that each step in the therapy should be explained and demonstrated to the mother so that she can understand and, as far as possible, participate in every phase of treatment. Thus when the child is for the first time beginning to use single words spontaneously, the mother will realize that if she tries to get him to say words at home she may inadvertently slow down his progress. A normal child can be encouraged and stimulated to attempt new words, but it may not be wise with a cerebral palsied child. The effort to respond may cause him to revert to his old pattern of motor behaviour so that the word is said, but in an abnormal way. In the initial stages of the treatment the mother will see that the therapist is careful to make no direct speech demands, and yet the situation is structured in such a way that the child spontaneously begins to use his few words for communication. Later on when he has more words, more confidence and greater experience of speaking, he will have to learn to speak on demand, and when attention is focussed on him, but this will only be in the final stages of the therapy.

GROUP THERAPY

No mention has yet been made of group therapy and the part it can play in the general habilitation picture. We believe that in the initial stages of the treatment (and with milder cases), it can be used for the *socialization* of the child, and in the later stages as part of his therapy. For example, in the initial stages a cerebral palsied child who is not too seriously handicapped needs to learn to be with other children and take part in shared play, or other activities. This situation can probably be handled best by the occupational therapist. At this stage, it would be quite impossible for cerebral palsied children to receive their physical, occupational or speech *therapy* in a group. As we have already described, each patient is evaluated individually, and the therapy is determined by his level of neuro-muscular development. Each child is likely to be at a different level of development, and so will require a different phase of the treatment. In addition, to inhibit or facilitate the required motor behaviour of *one* patient is quite as much as a therapist can handle.

At a much later stage of the treatment, however, when a patient has gained some voluntary control over more intricate movement patterns, the treatment might be given to a very small group of patients who have reached the same level. Specifically, from the point of view of the speech therapist, as soon as a child is able to say words voluntarily, and is beginning to combine them into short sentences, having one or two other children (at the same level of speech development) with him during the therapy session could be advantageous. It would create a more normal speech situation and help the child to carry over the type of speech he uses when alone with the speech therapist to the situations of everyday life. Obviously the situation would have to be carefully controlled or the children would become too excited and so revert to their former abnormal behaviour. This could only be harmful to them. With the emotional stimulation carefully graded and controlled by the therapist, it could raise the child's tolerance of disturbing outside influences, and so increase his chances of being able to speak in the normal situations of home life.

FUTURE TREATMENT OF THE CEREBRAL PALSIED CHILD

Our discussion of the cerebral palsied child cannot be concluded without some reference being made to the future, and what this could hold for him. We believe that the outstanding need of the present time is to separate cerebral palsied children from mentally retarded children. This need, of course, is recognized but, in our opinion, there are still far too many cerebral palsied children living in institutions for the mentally retarded.

The difficulties of assessing the intelligence of cerebral palsied children have already been mentioned, and are fully recognized. We feel that these children should be more carefully screened so that after initial assessments only the most obviously mentally retarded go to hospitals and schools for seriously retarded children. We believe that border line cases should be given the benefit of the doubt at least for several years.

As we have seen, a cerebral palsied child, as a result of his disabilities, inevitably develops both physically and mentally more slowly than the normal child, but innately he may have a normal intelligence. If during his early years he is treated as a normal (but slow developing) child, his mind may well develop; but, if during these years, he is surrounded by mentally retarded children, and is treated as such himself, it will not. The remedying of this situation is our first hope for the cerebral palsied child.

The second (closely related to it) is that the child should be given more treatment and less "custodial" care. Again, the need for this is recognized but, in our opinion, there are still too many cerebral palsied children attending centres where they are well-looked after and kept happy each day, but where they do not receive the treatment that they need. If effective therapy could also be given in these centres the child would have a better chance of fulfilling his potential.

Our third hope for the future is related to the treatment itself. We believe that the approach to cerebral palsy that we have described is, at the present time, the best that is available. This "holistic" approach is in keeping with the latest research on the working of the human body and mind, and our hope is that as further discoveries are made they will be related to the problem of the cerebral palsied child.

Our fourth hope is that, in the future, more attention will be directed to the cerebral palsied *adult*. In discussing this point, Wendell Johnson (53) writes: "There is at present a possibility that cerebral palsied children tend to be treated *as children* far beyond the age level at which they might better be dealt with as adults. If this is true, a major reason for it could be that no one has a very clear idea of the kind of adults most cerebral palsied children could, or should become." We believe that there is a great deal of truth in this. In our natural concern over cerebral palsied children we may not have prepared them sufficiently for their adult years; and this, in turn, may be largely due to the fact that we have not prepared a place for cerebral palsied *adults* in our society. For one thing, we have not given sufficient consideration to the question of their employment which, after all, is the basic factor in the lives of most adults. Therefore, our final hope is that local communities will make more provision for sheltered work-shops where cerebral palsied adults can learn to do some useful job. In some areas this has already been done, and sufficiently successfully to show that given the opportunity and work that is within their physical and mental capacities, the cerebral palsied adult is capable of producing good work. Many more such work-shops are needed, so that as the cerebral palsied child grows up he knows that there will be a place for him in society, and a job for him to do.

REFERENCES

1. ABBOTT, M.: *A Syllabus of Cerebral Palsy Treatment Techniques.* New York, United Cerebral Palsy, 1956.
2. ASHBY, W. R.: On the nature of inhibition: a review. *J. Ment. Sci., 80*:198, 1934.
3. BOBATH, B.: A study of abnormal postural reflex activity in patients with lesions of the CENTRAL nervous system. *Physiotherapy., 40*:9, 10, 11, 12, 1954.
4. BOBATH, K.: The treatment of cerebral palsy. *Spastics Quart., 2:3,* 1953.
5. BOBATH, K., and BOBATH, B.: An assessment of the motor handicap of children with cerebral palsy and of their response to treatment. *Occup. Ther. J., 21*:19, 1958.
6. BOBATH, K., and BOBATH, B.: Control of motor function in cerebral palsy. *Aust. J. Physiotherapy., 2*:75, 1958.
7. BOBATH, K., and BOBATH, B.: The diagnosis of cerebral palsy in infancy. *Dis. Child., 31*:408, 1956.
8. BOBATH, K., and BOBATH, B.: Spastic paralysis: treatment by the use of reflex inhibition. *Brit. J. Physical Med., 13*:121, 1950.
9. BOBATH, K., and BOBATH, B.: Tonic reflexes and righting reflexes in the diagnosis and assessment of cerebral palsy. *Cereb. Palsy Rev., 16*:4, 1955.
10. BOBATH, K., and BOBATH, B.: A treatment of cerebral palsy based on the analysis of the patient's motor behaviour. *Brit. J. Physical Med., 15*:107, 1952.
11. BOBATH, K., and BOBATH, B.: Treatment of cerebral palsy by the inhibition of abnormal reflex activity. *Brit. Orthoptic J., 11*:1, 1954.
12. BYRNE, M. C.: Speech and language development of athetoid and spastic children. *J.S.H.D., 24*:231, 1959.
13. CARLSON, E. R.: *Born That Way.* New York, Day, 1941.
14. CHUSID, J., and McDONALD, J.: *Correlative Neuroanatomy and Functional Neurology.* Los Altos, Lange, 1954.
15. CLEMENT, M., and TWITCHELL, T. E.: Dysarthria in cerebral palsy. *J.S.H.D., 24*:118, 1959.

16. COOPER, W.: The Clinic School. *Cerebral Palsy Proceedings.*, Project 194.
17. DARLEY, F. L., and WINITZ, H.: Age of the first word. *J.S.H.D.*, *26*:272, 1961.
18. DAWES, V. A.: Palatal dysfunction in cerebral palsy. Unpublished paper presented at A.S.H.A. convention, New York, 1958.
19. DENHOFF, E., and HOLDEN, R. H.: The significance of delayed development in the diagnosis of cerebral palsy. *J. Pediat.*, *38*:452, 1951.
20. DUFFEY, R. F.: An analysis of the pitch and duration characteristics of the speech of cerebral palsied individuals. Ph.D. Thesis, Purdue University, 1954.
21. ELLIS, G. E.: The interaction of the therapies and education of cerebral palsied children. *Conquering Physical Handicaps.*, Official proceedings of the first Pan-Pacific Conference, Sydney, 1958, p. 424.
22. EVANS, M. F.: Cerebral palsy. *Bull. Nat. Ass. of Secondary School Principals.*, *34*:63, 1950.
23. EVANS, M. F.: Problems in cerebral palsy. *J.S.D.*, *12*:87, 1947.
24. EVANS, M. F.: Techniques in speech rehabilitation for the cerebral palsied. *Speech Hearing Ther.*, December, 1951, p. 6.
25. FAIRGRIEVES, E.: Occupational therapy and the Bobath approach to cerebral palsy. An unpublished study, 1963.
26. FLETCHER, S. A., CASTEEL, R. L., and BRADLEY, D. P.: Tongue-thrust, swallow, speech articulation and age. *J.S.H.D.*, *26*:201, 1961.
27. GESELL, A.: *Infant Development.* New York, Harper, 1952.
28. GESELL, A., and ARMATRUDA, C. S.: *Developmental Diagnosis.* London, Hoeber, 1949.
29. GESELL, A., and ILG, F.: *Infant and Child in the Culture Today.* New York and London, Harper, 1943.
30. GESELL, A., and THOMPSON, H.: *Infant Behaviour: Its Genesis and Growth.* New York and London, McGraw-Hill, 1934.
31. GOLDSCHMIDT, P.: De behandeling van de spastiche paralyse volgens, Bobath. *Logopaedie Int. Phonatrie.*, *25*:18, 34, and 51, 1953.
32. GOLDSCHMIDT, P., and GESELL, A.: Language and speech development from birth onward. Unpublished study.
33. GRATKE, J. M.: Speech problems of the cerebral palsied. *J.S.D.*, *12*:129, 1947.
34. GREENE, M. C.: *Learning to Talk.* New York and London, Harper,

1960.

35. GRIFFITHS, R.: *The Abilities of Babies.* New York and London, McGraw-Hill, 1954.

36. HAHN, E. F.: A discussion of the moto-kinesthetic method of speech correction. *Quart. J. Speech., 25:*417, 1939.

37. HARDY, J. C.: Intraoral breath pressure in cerebral palsy. *J.S.H.D., 26:*309, 1961.

38. HAWK, S. STINCHFIELD: Moto-kinesthetic speech training for Children. *J.S.H.D., 2:*230, 1937.

39. HELTMAN, J. H., and PEACHER, G. M.: Mis-articulation and diadochokinesis in the spastic paralytic. *J.S.H.D., 8:*137, 1943.

40. HIPPS, H. E.: Basic teacher training principles for the patient with cerebral palsy. *Amer. J. Surg., 91:*715, 1956.

41. HOBERMAN, S. L., and HOBERMAN, M.: Speech habilitation in cerebral palsy. *J.S.H.D., 25:*111, 1960.

42. HOOD, P. N., and PERLSTEIN, M. A.: Infantile spastic hemiplegia. *Pediatrics., 17:*58, 1956.

43. HOOD, P. N., SHANK, K. H., and WILLIAMSON, D. B.: Environmental factors in relation to the speech of cerebral palsied children. *J.S.H.D., 13:*325, 1948.

44. HOPKINS, T. W., BICE, A. V., and COLTON, K. G.: *Evaluation and Education of the Cerebral Palsied Child: New Jersey Study.* Washington, D. C., I.C.E.C., 1954.

45. HUBER, M.: Letter to the parents of the cerebral palsied child. *J.S.H.D., 15:*154, 1950.

46. HURLOCK, E. B.: *Child Development.* New York, McGraw-Hill, 1950.

47. IRWIN, O. C.: Infant speech: development of vowel sounds. *J.S.H.D., 13:*31, 1948.

48. IRWIN, O. C.: *Language and Communication.* New York, Wiley, 1960.

49. IRWIN, O. C.: Phonetic equipment of spastic and athetoid children. *J.S.H.D., 20:*54, 1955.

50. IRWIN, O. C.: Research on speech sounds for the first six months of life. *Psychol. Bull., 38:*277, 1941.

51. JACOBSON, E.: *Progressive Relaxation.* Chicago, Univ. Chicago Press, 1929.

52. JENKINS, R. E.: The rate of diadochokinetic movement of the jaw at the ages from seven to maturity. *J.S.D., 6:*13, 1941.

53. JOHNSON, W.: Adjustment problems of the cerebral palsied. *J.S.H.D., 21:*12, 1956.

54. KABAT, H., and KNOTT, M.: Proprioceptive facilitation techniques for treatment of paralysis. *Physical Ther. Rev.*, *33*:53, 1953.

55. KOSTER, S.: The diagnosis of disorders of occlusion in children with cerebral palsy. *J. Dent. Child.*, *23*:81, 1956.

56. LEITH, W., and STEER, M. D.: Comparison of judged speech characteristics of athetoids and spastics. *Cereb. Palsy Rev.*, *19*:15, 1958.

57. MARLAND, P. M.: Speech therapy for the cerebral palsied based on reflex inhibition. *Speech.*, *17*:65, 1953.

58. McCARTHY, D.: Language development of the pre-school child. Institute of Child Welfare Monograph, Series 4. Univ. Minnesota Press, 1930.

59. MITCHELL, J.: Communication disorders following cerebral lesions: the team approach in rehabilitation. *Speech Path. Ther.*, *6*:54, 1963.

60. MORLEY, M. E.: *The development of Disorders of Speech In Childhood.* London, Livingstone, 1957.

61. MOWRER, O. H.: Hearing and speaking; an analysis of language learning. *J.S.H.D.*, *23*:143, 1957.

62. MUYSKENS, J. H.: The smallest aggregate of speech analysed and defined: the hypha. *Doctoral dissertation. Univ. Michigan*, 1931.

63. MYSAK, E. D.: Organismic development of oral language. *J.S.H.D.*, *26*:377, 1961.

64. MYSAK, E. D.: Significance of neurophysiological orientation to cerebral palsy habilitation. *J.S.H.D.*, *24*:221, 1959.

65. NEAL, HELEN: *Better Communications for Better Health.* National Health Forum. New York, Columbia Univ. Press, 1962.

66. PALMER, M. F.: Similarities of the effects of environmental pressures on cerebral palsy and stuttering. *J.S.H.D.*, *8*:150, 1943.

67. PALMER, M. F.: Studies in clinical techniques. *J.S.H.D.*, *12*:415, 1947.

68. PENFIELD, W., and ROBERTS, L.: *Speech and Brain Mechanisms.* Princeton, Princeton Univ. Press, 1959.

69. PERLSTEIN, M.: *Cerebral Palsy.* Chicago, National Society for Crippled Children and Adults, Parent series No. 9, 1961.

70. PHELPS, W. M.: Description and differentiation of types of cerebral palsy. *Nervous Child.*, *8*:107, 1949.

71. PIAGET, J.: *The Language and Thought of the Child.* London, Routledge, 1948.

72. Pintner, R., Eisenson, J., and Stanton, M.: *The Psychology of the Physically Handicapped.* New York, Crofts, 1941.

73. Rood, M.: Neurophysiological reactions as a basis for physical therapy. *Physical Ther. Rev., 34*:444, 1954.

74. Ruch, C. H.: *Psychology and Life.* Chicago, Scott, Foresman, 1952.

75. Rutherford, B.: A comparative study of loudness, pitch, rate, rhythm and quality of the speech of children handicapped by cerebral palsy. *J.S.H.D., 9*:263, 1944.

76. Schaltenbrand, G.: Some observations on development of human motility and on motor disturbances. *Bull. N. Y. Acad. Med., 3*:534, 1927.

77. Schlanger, B. B.: A longitudinal study of brain damaged retarded children. *J.S.H.D., 24*:354, 1959.

78. Shelton, R. L., Jr., Arndt, W. B. Jr., and Miller, J. B.: Learning principles and teaching of speech language. *J.S.H.D., 26*: 368, 1961.

79. Sherrington, C. S.: *The Integrative Action of the Nervous System.* Cambridge, Cambridge Univ. Press, 1947.

80. Sittig, E.: The chewing method applied for excessive salivation and drooling in cerebral palsy. *J.S.H.D., 12*:194, 1947.

81. Straub, W. J.: Malfunction of the tongue. *Amer. J. Orthondont., 46*:404, 1960.

82. Van Riper, C.: *Speech Correction—Principles and Methods.* 3rd Ed. New York, Prentice-Hall, 1954.

83. Van Riper, C.: *Speech Correction—Principles and Methods.* 4th Ed. Englewood Cliffs, Prentice-Hall, 1963.

84. Van Riper, C.: *Teaching Your Child To Talk.* New York, Harper, 1950.

85. Van Riper, C., and Irwin, J.: *Voice and Articulation.* Englewood Cliffs, Prentice-Hall, 1958.

86. Ward, M., Malone, Sister H., Jann, G., and Jann, H. W.: Articulation variations associated with visceral swallowing and malocclusion. *J.S.H.D., 26*:334, 1961.

87. Westlake, H., and Rutherford, D.: *Speech for the Cerebral Palsied.* Chicago, National Society for Crippled Children and Adults, 1961.

88. Wilson, F. B.: The effect of a superimposed respiratory pattern on the breathing and speech of eight athetoid children. *Ph.D. Thesis.* Northwestern University, 1958.

89. Wolfe, W. A.: A comprehensive evaluation of fifty cases of cerebral palsy. *J.S.H.D., 15*:234, 1950.

90. Wyllie, W. G.: *The Cerebral Palsies of Childhood*. London, Butterworth, 1951.
91. Young, E. Hill, and Hawk, S. Stinchfield: *Moto-kinesthetic Speech Training*. Stanford Univ. Press, 1958.

INDEX